The Smile Diet
Eat Right & Smile Bright

The key to a radiant smile is on your plate —unlock the power of natural, smile—friendly foods!

by Mason Preddy

First Edition 2025

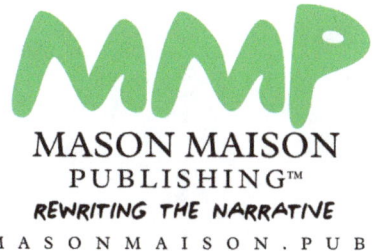

MASON MAISON PUBLISHING™
REWRITING THE NARRATIVE
M A S O N M A I S O N . P U B

Dedication

To my mom, **Garland Preddy**—

For always being the calm in my chaos, the laughter in my disasters, and the co-pilot (literally and figuratively) in some of the most ridiculous adventures life has thrown my way.

Your unwavering support and your own radiant smile have always been the guiding light in my life, inspiring me to help others find their own.

This book—and every smile it creates—is because of you.

Always 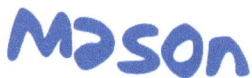 !

I love you.

Mason

The Smile Diet

Eat Right & Smile Bright

© 2025 by Mason Preddy.

Published by Mason Maison Publishing™
490 M ST SW W602
Washington, DC 20024-2628, USA

No part of this publication may be reproduced, distributed, or transmitted, storied in a retrieval system, or transmitted in any form or any means— electronic, mechanical, photocopied, recorded, or otherwise— without the prior written permission of the publisher, except for brief quotations used in reviews, articles, or academic references.

For permissions, we welcome you to reach out to us at vip@masonmaison.pub.

This book is a work of non-fiction. While every effort has been made to ensure the accuracy of the content, the author and publisher make no representations or warranties regarding the completeness, reliability, or accuracy of the information contained herein. The advice and strategies presented are intended for informational purposes only and should not be considered as professional, legal or career counseling. Readers should consult a qualified professional for advice tailored to their specific situation.

The author and publisher disclaim and liability, loss, or risk incurred as a direct or indirect consequence of the use and application of any contents of this book.

First Edition: April 2025

Printed in the United States of America

All rights reserved.

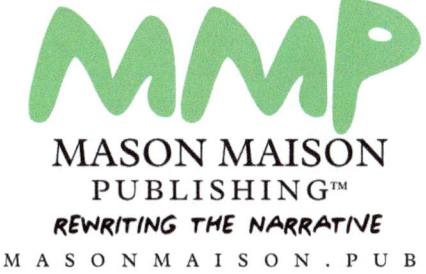

MASON MAISON
PUBLISHING™
REWRITING THE NARRATIVE
MASONMAISON.PUB

Table of Contents

Foreword 9
Preface..11
Introduction..13

A..17
Almonds 18
Aloe Vera...18
Apples 19
Apple Cider Vinegar 20
Artichokes 21
Avocados...21

B..22
Baking Soda 23
1. Baking Soda and Lemon Juice..................................23
3. Baking Soda and Hydrogen Peroxide 24
2. Baking Soda and Coconut Oil 24
5. Baking Soda and Water 25
4. Baking Soda and Strawberry...................................25
Balsamic Vinegar 26
Bananas 27
Basil..28
Beets...29
Bell Peppers...29

Beverages 30
The Science of Seltzer Water...31
Sparkling Water 32
Club Soda..33
Tonic Water..34
Energy Drinks 35
Sports Drinks 36
Alcoholic Beverages 37
Coffee...39
Tea 41
Regular Iced Tea...43
Sweetened Iced Tea..44
Red vs. White Wine 45
Fruit Juices...47
Cola and Diet Cola...49
Cola 49

Diet Cola 50
Flavored Water & Vitamin Waters 51
Flavored Water 51
Vitamin Waters 51
Milkshakes and Smoothies 53
Milkshakes 53

Smoothies.. 54
Blackberries..55
Blueberries...56
Bok Choy..57
Broccoli...58
Brussels Sprouts 59

C... 60
Cabbage 61
Cherries...62
Cranberries...63
Cucumbers 64
Candy 65
Cauliflower 66
Carrots..67
Celery..68
Crafting a Tooth-Friendly Charcuterie Board..69
1. Start with Cheese 69
2. Add Your Meats 70
3. Veggies..70
4. Fruit..70
5. Healthy Dips 70
6. Whole Grains...71
7. Nutrient-Rich Nuts 71
8. Unhealthy Additions to Avoid...71
9. Build Your Board 71
Cheese 72
Citrus Squeeze...74
Citrus Lemon 76
Cinnamon 77
Clove...79
Cocoa 80
Coffee and Tea 81

D 82
The Dairy Defense 83

E **84**
Edamame 85
Echinacea 87
Eggs 89
Endive 90

F **92**
Figs 93
Fish 94

G **95**
Garlic 96
Ginger Root 97
Grapes 98
Green Tea 99
Green Beans 100
Guava 101
GUM 102
Nibble Knowledge 103
Gummy Vitamins 104

H **105**
Herbs 106
Honey 108
Hummus 110
Hydrogen Peroxide 112
Hydrate for Health 115

I **116**
ICE 117
Iron Supplements 119

J **120**
Juice 121

K **122**
Kale 123
Kiwi 124
Kombucha 126

L **128**
Lavender 129
Leafy Greens 131
Lettuce 132

Limes..133

M..134
Matcha..135
Medications That Can Stain Teeth 137
Got Milk?..138
Miso 139
Mint Leaves...141
Melons 142
Mushrooms...144

N..146
Nectarines...147
Neem 149
Nuts...150

O..151
Oil Pulling..152
Olives 155
Onions..156
Orange 158

P..160
Papayas..161
Parsley..162
Peas...163
Peaches..164
Pears...165
Peppers..166
Pineapple..167
The Power of Smiling 168

R..170
Radishes..171
Raisins..172
Raspberries...173
Rhubarb...174

S..176
Sage..177
Sauces..178
Seeds..179
Shiitake Mushrooms 180
Smoking..181

Spices 182
Sip and Smile 183
Seaweed 185
Sesame 186
Strawberries 187
Sugary Drinks 189

T **190**
Turmeric 191
Tomatoes 192
Turnips 193

U **194**
Udon Noodles 195

V **196**
Extra Virgin Olive Oil 197

W **198**
Walnuts 199
WATER 200
Watermelon 201
Wine 204

Y **208**
Yogurt 209

Z **210**
Zucchini 211

TIPS 215

Foreword

I first met Mason as a child, when he was a patient in my dental practice in Northern Virginia. Little did I know, years later, that I would become his first client when he was just 13 years old, taking care of our saltwater aquarium in the reception area of my practice. Mason had started a business selling and taking care of saltwater aquariums for businesses in the Washington, DC suburbs, and we were his very first client. Over the years, our families continued to stay connected. Our sons, Marc, and Pete, even attended Fork Union Military Academy together. Fast forward a few more years, and once again, my wife Mary and I had the pleasure of being his first clients in his mobile dry-cleaning business, Pressed 4 Time. Watching Mason grow from a bright young man into a successful entrepreneur has been a joy and a testament to his work ethic, dedication, and commitment to excellence. So, it only seems fitting that this "serial entrepreneur" would ask me to write the foreword to his book, another chapter in his impressive journey.

Welcome to The Smile Diet, where the power of your plate meets the brilliance of your smile! This is a book about one of your most powerful assets—your smile. Everything you eat or drink can impact your smile. We often hear that a smile is the best accessory you can wear, but did you know that what you eat can make your smile shine even brighter? This book is here to show you how the foods you choose can affect not just your overall health but the radiance of your smile too.

Over the years, we've learned that a glowing smile isn't just about brushing, flossing, and whitening treatments. It's about understanding the connection between what we consume and the health of our teeth and gums.

As you read through these pages, you'll discover foods that can naturally brighten your teeth, others that will do the opposite, and herbs that support oral health—keeping your smile gleaming for years to come. But this book isn't just about what to eat; it's about how to enjoy the journey to a whiter, brighter, and healthier smile. You'll find recipes, tips, and insights that make caring for your teeth a delicious and rewarding experience.

You're in the right place. In this guide, we're diving into the world of oral health, exploring how the foods you consume daily can either be your smile's best friend or its sneaky foe.

Let's face it, food is an essential part of our lives. It fuels us, comforts us, and brings us together. But did you know that every bite you take has the potential to affect your teeth? Yes, it's true! All food can leave enamel-eating plaque on your teeth, turning your mouth into a battleground for your oral health.

However, it's not all doom and gloom. Some foods can be harmful, but others are packed with essential vitamins and minerals that support and strengthen your teeth and gums. Imagine eating your way to a whiter, brighter, and healthier smile—it sounds delicious, doesn't it?

In The Smile Diet, you'll uncover the best and worst foods for your teeth. From the acidic villains that erode your enamel to the vitamin-packed heroes that strengthen your gums, you'll learn how to make smarter dietary choices that benefit not only your overall health but also enhance your smile.

So whether you're here to learn how to keep your pearly whites at their best or simply to explore how food can impact your oral health, The Smile Diet is your go-to guide. May your smile become even more radiant with every bite!

Peter J. Repole, **DMD, FAGD**

PREFACE

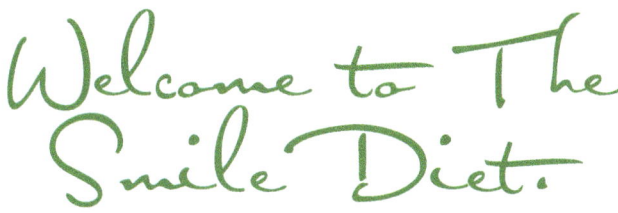
Welcome to The Smile Diet.

I am excited to embark on this journey with you towards a whiter, brighter, healthier smile.

First things first. Don't worry, I'm not here to lecture you about eating and drinking stain-causing foods. I'm not your dentist, I'm not even a dentist. I'm just your friendly reminder that bacteria love some of these things as much as you do—maybe even more.

I'm here to share with you what I have learned through the years when it comes to the various types of staining agents and how they affect your teeth.

At WhiteBrights®, we understand the importance of a radiant smile. Not only for its aesthetic appeal but also for its impact on overall confidence and well-being.

The Smile Diet is more than just a dietary guide—it's a holistic approach to oral health and teeth whitening. What you eat plays a significant role in the health and appearance of your smile.

With the right foods and nutrients, you can enhance the natural brightness of your teeth while promoting strong, healthy gums and maintaining optimal oral hygiene.

Concentrating on your oral health now can save you tens of thousands of dollars down the road.

In this book, we'll study the science behind The Smile Diet, exploring the foods and beverages that can help you achieve a dazzling smile while also supporting your overall health. From nutrient-rich fruits and vegetables to teeth-friendly snacks, we'll provide practical tips and delicious recipes to incorporate into your daily routine.

Join us as we discover the power of nutrition in unlocking your brightest smile yet. Let's nourish our smiles from within and radiate confidence with every grin. Welcome to The Smile Diet—it's time to smile whiter, brighter, and healthier.

Stay Smilin!

Mason Preddy

Mason Preddy, CHCR, CDR, CIR
Founder/CEO
WhiteBrights®

INTRODUCTION

Welcome to The *Smile Diet*, where we believe that your smile is as much a reflection of your diet as it is of your personality.

Imagine a world where every bite you take not only satisfies your taste buds but also brightens your smile. Well, that's the world we're creating right here, right now!

The *Smile Diet* isn't just another book about healthy eating—it's a culinary journey to a whiter, brighter, and healthier smile. We're all about smart, delicious choices that help you shine from the inside out, making every smile a little more dazzling.

At my cosmetic oral cosmetics company, WhiteBrights®, we've spent years perfecting the art and science of teeth whitening, and now we're excited to share how the right foods can complement our products, giving you even more reasons to smile. Whether you're a foodie or just looking to improve your oral health, this guide is packed with tips, recipes, and fun facts that'll have you grinning from ear to ear.

But don't worry—we're not here to tell you to give up everything you love. Instead, we're here to show you how small, tasty changes can make a big impact on your smile and your overall well-being.

From the best foods to boost your pearly whites to those you might want to enjoy in moderation, we've got you covered.

So, let's get started on this delicious journey. After all, a brighter smile is just a bite away!

Eat Right & Smile Bright

> *The key to a radiant smile is on your plate—unlock the power of natural smile-friendly foods!*

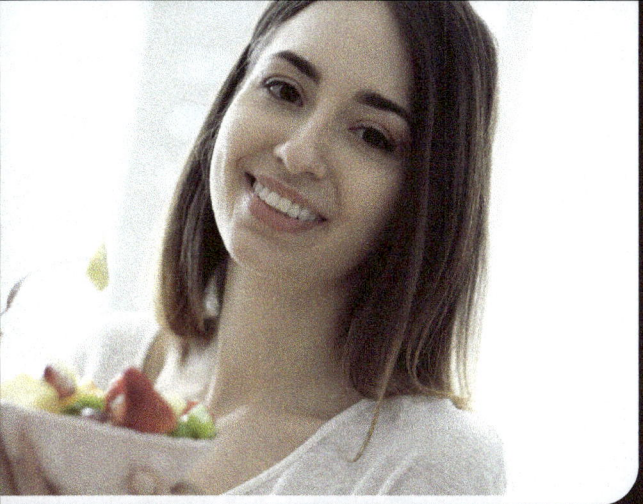

Foods That Whiten Teeth Naturally Affordable Home Remedies That Work

While coffee, tea, red wine, and some sodas can stain your teeth, there are common foods that can help whiten them over time.

Though not as effective as professional whitening products, these natural and inexpensive options can still brighten your smile—and that's something to smile about!

Delve into the enchanting world of smiles and discover their incredible ability to brighten your day. Whether it's a mischievous smirk, a gentle grin, a dazzling beam, or a serene smile, each holds boundless potential to lift your mood and elevate your spirits.

> *I genuinely believe that if we all smiled a little more, the world would shine a whole lot brighter.*
>
> *- Mason Preddy*

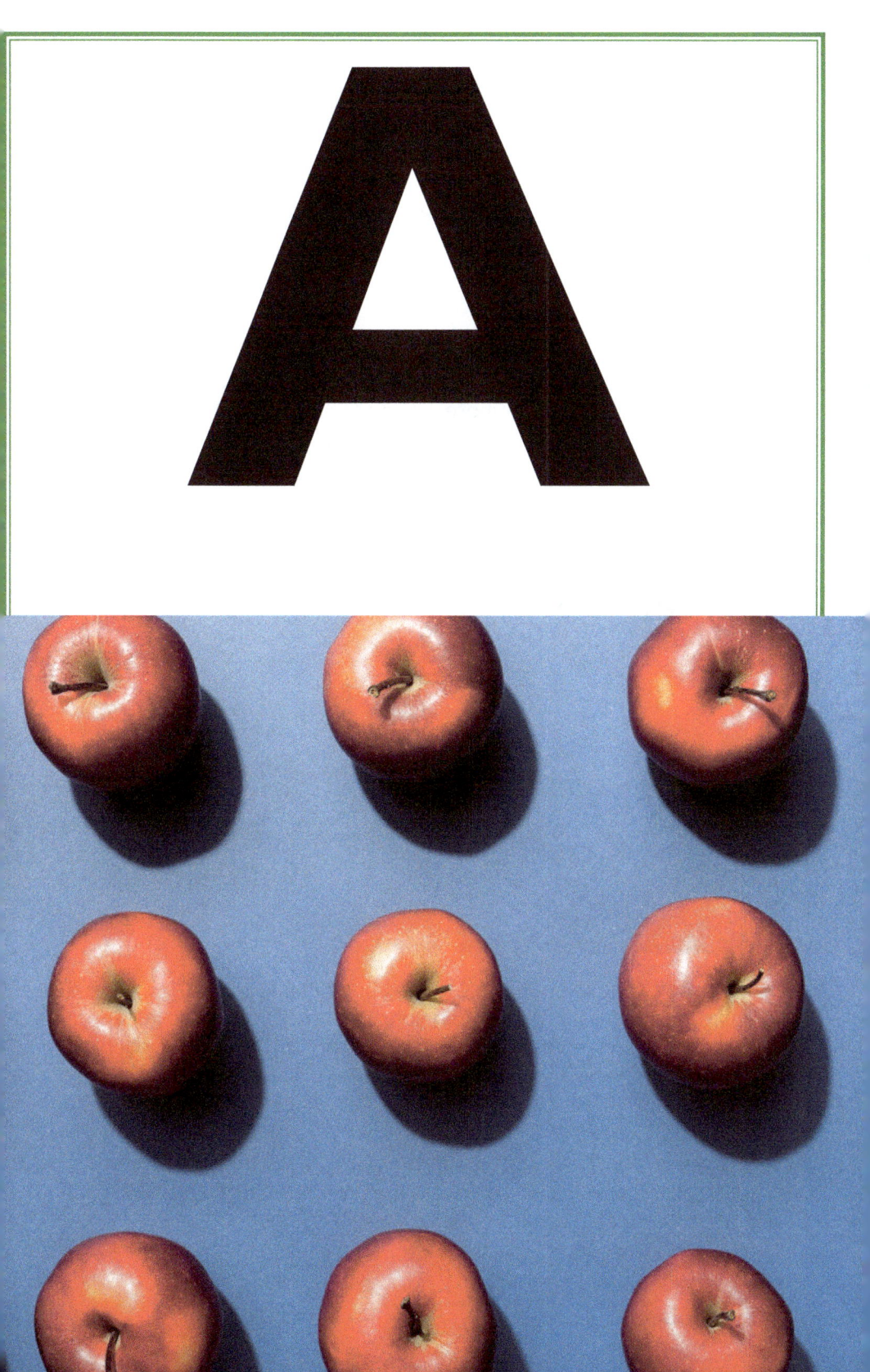

Almonds

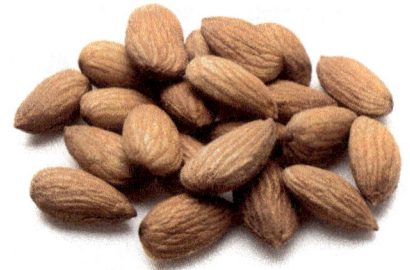

Crunch Your Way to a Brighter Smile

Almonds aren't just a nutritious snack—they're also a natural way to help whiten your teeth. Rich in protein, healthy fats, and essential nutrients, almonds provide more than just a health boost. Their crunchy texture acts like a natural toothbrush, helping to scrub away stains and plaque from your teeth. Additionally, almonds are high in calcium, which is vital for maintaining strong, healthy enamel. Incorporating almonds into your diet can contribute to a brighter, whiter smile while also supporting overall oral health. Snack on a handful of almonds daily and enjoy the dual benefits of a healthier body and a naturally radiant smile!

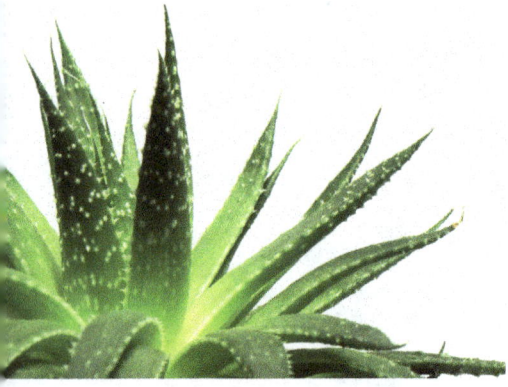

Aloe Vera

Your Natural Teeth Whitener

Aloe vera is renowned for its soothing and healing properties, but did you know it can also help whiten your teeth naturally? The gel inside aloe vera leaves contains compounds that not only fight bacteria but also help remove stains from your teeth. By reducing plaque and fighting gum inflammation, aloe vera promotes overall oral health, which contributes to a whiter smile. Simply use aloe vera gel as a natural toothpaste or rinse your mouth with aloe vera juice to reap its benefits. Incorporating aloe vera into your oral hygiene routine is a gentle and effective way to achieve a brighter, healthier smile.

Apples

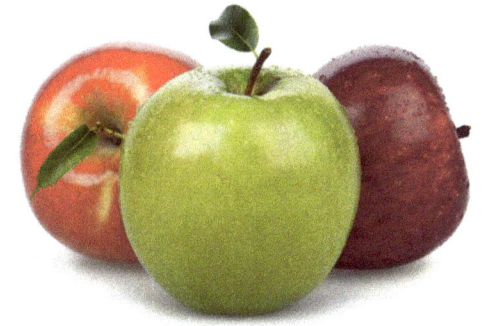

Munching and Crunching

That loud crunch you hear when you bite into an apple is actually helping to strengthen your gums, and the fruit's high water content increases saliva production. These crunchy fruits work as a natural abrasive scrub for your teeth when you chomp on them.

Apples have long been called "nature's toothbrush," and for good reason. They have a crisp texture and firm skin that scrape away plaque and the bacteria that cause it. Apples' tangy flavor combines with the texture to stimulate saliva production.

Saliva serves as your mouth's self-cleaning agent and as your mouth's natural defense against decay and staining.

If you're searching for one of the best foods for whiter teeth, you don't have to look any further than apples. This nutritious fruit is one of the best stain-fighting natural foods available.

> An apple a day keeps the dentist away.

Apple Cider Vinegar

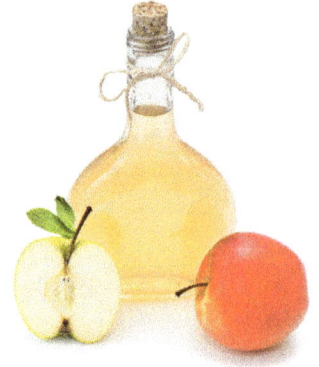

Swish, Swish, Give Your Mouth a Bath!

Apple cider vinegar is very effective for getting rid of stains on your teeth.

Swish it around your teeth at full strength, if you can tolerate it! Or you can try brushing your teeth with a tablespoon of apple cider vinegar to help remove stains, and then gargle with a mouthful to help freshen your breath and kill bacteria around your gums.

You can also mix apple cider vinegar with baking soda. This mixture can be rubbed on the teeth like a polish. Be easy though, using too much of this formula can and probably will cause tooth sensitivity.

While it might not be the most glamorous thought, that extra bit of saliva in your mouth produces a natural defense mechanism. It helps wash away bacteria that could lead to discoloration, keeping your smile bright. Some foods help your body produce more saliva than others and we'll be talking about those.

And don't forget the power of water! If you can't brush after eating, rinsing with water is a simple yet effective way to wash away debris and keep your teeth clean between meals.

Artichokes

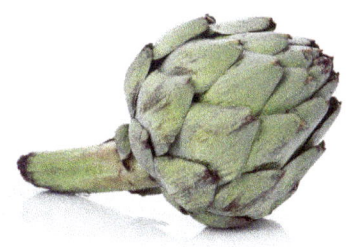

A Delicious Path to Whiter Teeth

Artichokes are more than just a tasty addition to your meals—they can also help whiten your teeth naturally. These fiber-rich vegetables promote saliva production, which is essential for washing away food particles and bacteria that can cause stains. The increased saliva flow helps to neutralize acids in the mouth, protecting enamel and preventing discoloration. Additionally, artichokes are packed with vitamins and antioxidants that support overall oral health. Adding artichokes to your diet is a delicious way to contribute to a brighter, whiter smile while enjoying their numerous health benefits.

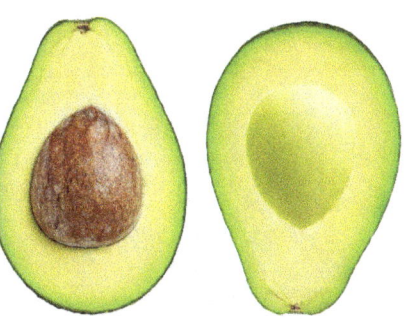

Avocados

The Creamy Secret to a Whiter Smile

Avocados aren't just a superfood for your body—they're also great for your teeth! Rich in healthy fats, vitamins, and minerals, avocados help promote overall oral health. Their high fiber content stimulates saliva production, which naturally cleanses your teeth and helps prevent staining. Additionally, avocados contain potassium and magnesium, which support strong enamel and protect against tooth decay. Incorporating avocados into your diet not only boosts your health but also contributes to a naturally brighter, whiter smile.

> ❝
> *Enjoy this creamy delight and let your smile shine!*
> ❞

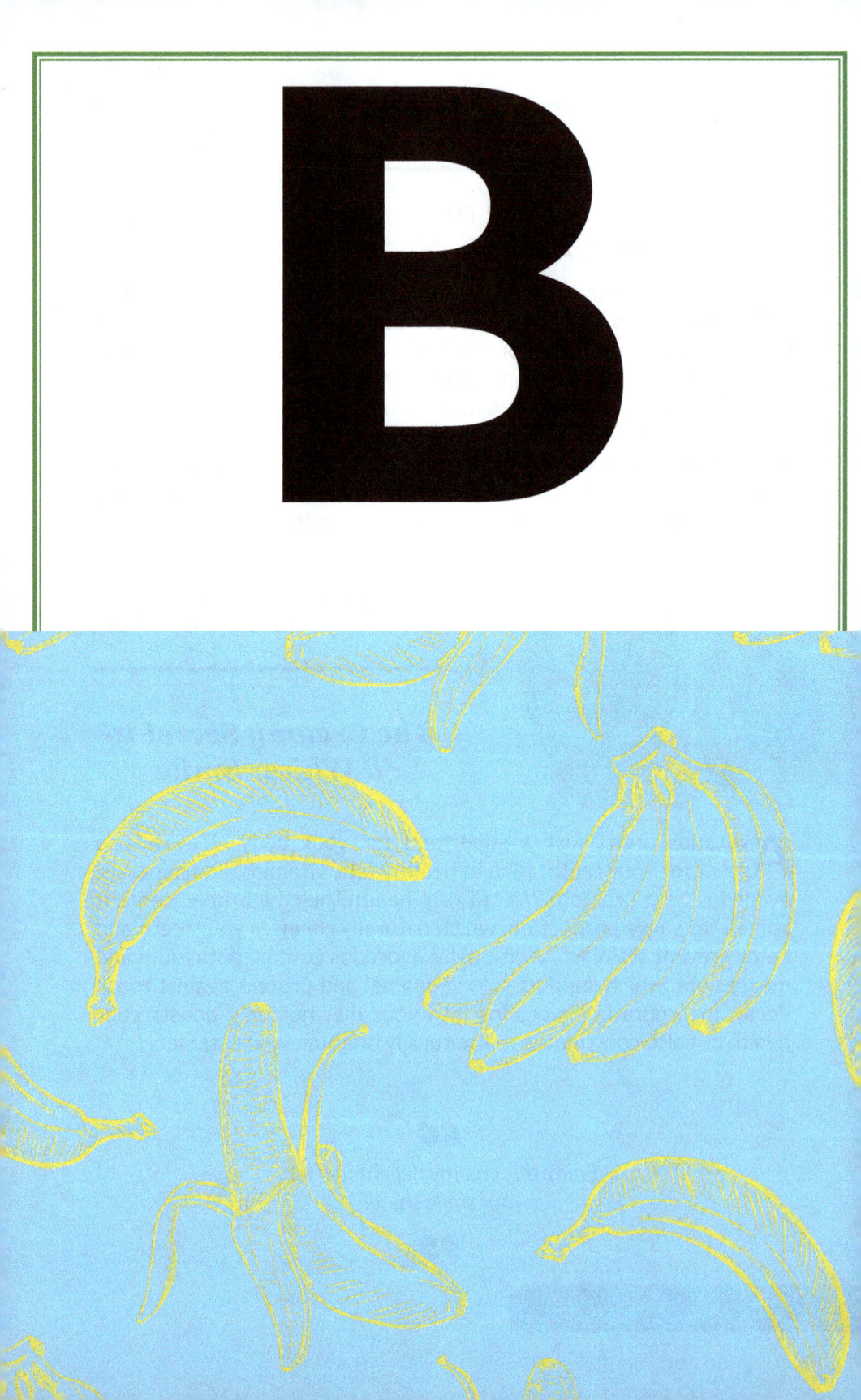

Baking Soda

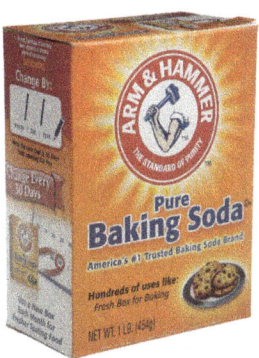

It's the oldest DIY whitening remedy in the book.

Once in a while, it is OK to add a dash of baking soda to your toothpaste for its mild abrasive properties when used in moderation. Baking soda can help polish teeth and remove surface stains.

I personally like to create a paste in the palm of my hand. Here's how to do it:

Wash your hands. Sprinkle some Baking Soda from the box into the palm of your hands. Lightly flick some water in your hand and make a circular action, creating a paste in the palm of your hand. Dip your toothbrush in your mixture and brush as normal.

Be careful though. Baking soda is a very abrasive material. Prolonged use of this type of hack may cause tooth sensitivity and even damage your enamel.

1. Baking Soda and Lemon Juice

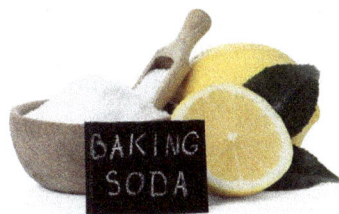

A Powerful Duo for a Brighter Smile

Baking soda and lemon juice create a potent natural teeth-whitening paste. Baking soda is a mild abrasive that gently removes surface stains and plaque from your teeth, while its alkaline properties help neutralize acids in the mouth. Lemon juice, rich in citric acid, enhances this effect by breaking down stains and whitening teeth.To use, mix a small amount of baking soda with fresh lemon juice to form a paste, apply it to your teeth, and leave it on for a minute before rinsing thoroughly. Be sure to use this mixture sparingly, as the acidity of lemon juice can weaken enamel if overused. Incorporate this powerful duo into your oral care routine for a brighter, whiter smile naturally!

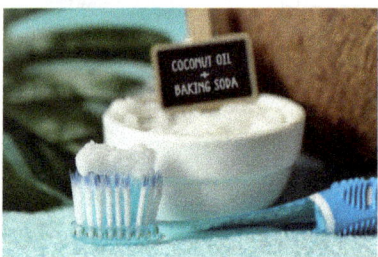

2. Baking Soda and Coconut Oil

A Natural Combo for a Radiant Smile

Baking soda and coconut oil combine to create an effective, natural teeth-whitening paste. Baking soda's mild abrasive properties help remove surface stains and plaque, while its alkaline nature neutralizes harmful acids in the mouth. Coconut oil adds its antibacterial and anti-inflammatory benefits, promoting overall oral health.To use, mix a small amount of baking soda with coconut oil to form a paste, apply it to your teeth, and brush gently for a minute before rinsing thoroughly. Incorporating this natural combo into your oral care routine can help you achieve a brighter, whiter smile while keeping your teeth and gums healthy. Enjoy the dual benefits of a radiant smile and improved oral health!

3. Baking Soda and Hydrogen Peroxide

A Dynamic Duo for a Whiter Smile

Combining baking soda and hydrogen peroxide creates a powerful natural teeth-whitening paste. Baking soda's mild abrasiveness helps scrub away surface stains and plaque, while its alkaline properties neutralize acids in the mouth. Hydrogen peroxide, a natural bleaching agent, works to break down stains and whiten teeth effectively. To use, mix a small amount of baking soda with a few drops of hydrogen peroxide to form a paste, apply it to your teeth, and brush gently for a minute before rinsing thoroughly. This dynamic duo can help you achieve a brighter, whiter smile naturally, while also maintaining your overall oral health.

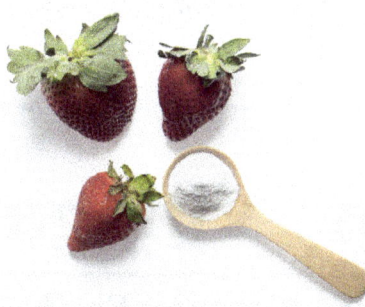

4. Baking Soda and Strawberry

A Sweet Solution for a Whiter Smile

Baking soda and strawberries team up to create a deliciously effective natural teeth-whitening paste. Baking soda's gentle abrasiveness helps to remove surface stains and plaque, while strawberries contain malic acid, a natural enzyme that helps break down and dissolve stains. To use, mash a ripe strawberry and mix it with a small amount of baking soda to form a paste. Apply this mixture to your teeth, leave it on for a few minutes, then rinse thoroughly and brush with regular toothpaste. Incorporating this sweet solution into your oral care routine can help you achieve a brighter, whiter smile naturally, while also enjoying the refreshing taste of strawberries.

5. Baking Soda and Water

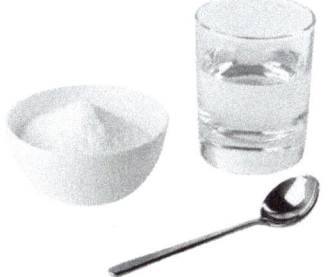

A Simple Solution for a Whiter Smile

Baking soda and water create an easy and effective natural teeth whitening paste. Baking soda's mild abrasive properties help remove surface stains and plaque, while its alkaline nature neutralizes acids in the mouth. To use, mix a small amount of baking soda with water to form a paste, apply it to your teeth, and brush gently for a minute before rinsing thoroughly. This simple solution can be incorporated into your oral care routine to help you achieve a brighter, whiter smile naturally. Enjoy the benefits of a radiant smile with just two common household ingredients!

Balsamic Vinegar

Skip the Sour, Keep the Smile

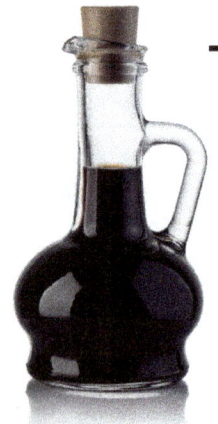

While great on a salad, it creates havoc on your teeth. If you must, enjoy it "lightly" on lettuce. Doing so will provide a protective film over your teeth. However, due to its natural color and acidic content Balsamic vinegar can also darken your teeth. This can encourage staining from other foods. Eating raw, crunchy veggies with balsamic vinegar will help, but be sure to brush shortly afterward for best results.

Bananas

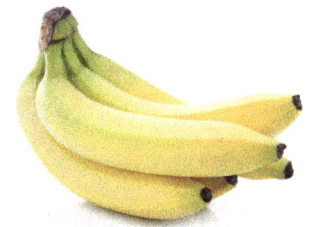

Peel away the myths: Unveiling the surprising truth about bananas and your smile!

Bananas have plenty of minerals and nutrients that are good for your teeth. Bananas provide a wide variety of minerals like potassium, manganese, and magnesium. These minerals can help strengthen your tooth enamel, so they're very good for your teeth. Overall, they are a very healthy food.

Be Aware, Bananas Are Also High In Starch And Sugars

Even though they're good for you, most fruits like bananas have high sugar content. Just like sugar from any other source, this sugar can contribute to tooth decay.

Bananas are also pretty gummy and starchy, which means they're more likely to stick to your teeth. This can also contribute to a higher risk of tooth decay.

However, these negative aspects of bananas can easily be controlled with proper dental hygiene. As long as you're brushing your teeth properly and consuming a healthy diet with a reasonable amount of sugar, eating a banana per day won't have any negative effects on your teeth.

Banana Peel Teeth Whitening? Don't slip up and monkey around!

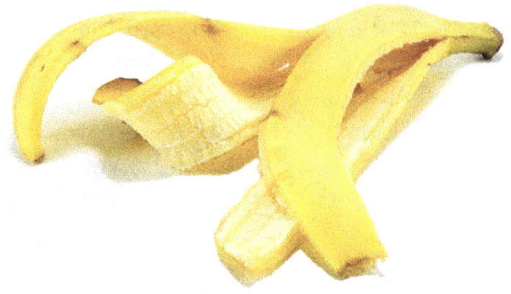

Banana peels do not have anything to do with whitening your teeth. lol. While you may have seen it posted, shared, or blogged, when it comes to whitening or removing stains from your teeth, there are no scientific studies that say banana peels are up to the job.

The American Dental Association (ADA) doesn't weigh in on using banana peels to whiten teeth, but they do have strong opinions on other fruit-based methods, like strawberries, orange peels, and lemons.

Their advice? Steer clear. While fruits are great for your diet, using them to whiten your teeth can backfire. The high acidity in many fruits can actually damage your teeth instead of brightening them. If you're looking to enhance your smile, skip the banana peel and opt for a teeth whitening option that is a safe, and effective whitening option.

Basil

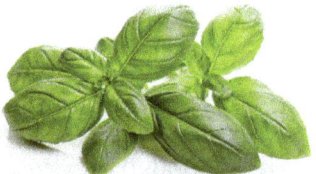

Not just for pasta - Discover its surprising benefits for your teeth and smile.

Harness the power of basil, renowned for its potent natural antibiotic properties. By incorporating basil into your oral care routine, you can effectively decrease the presence of harmful bacteria in the mouth. Basil acts as a formidable defense mechanism, not only reducing bacteria levels but also thwarting their proliferation.

Experience the Magic of Basil for Teeth Whitening

Discover a simple yet effective method for at-home teeth whitening by harnessing the power of basil. Crush dried basil leaves into a fine powder, creating a mildly abrasive substance. Mix this powder with mustard oil, known for its antibacterial, anti-fungal, and anti-inflammatory properties, for a fast and efficient whitening solution. Alternatively, utilize fresh basil leaves by crushing them into WhiteBrights® TwinPower® Teeth Whitening Foam or a toothpaste and apply directly onto your teeth using a toothbrush.

Basil not only aids in teeth whitening but also serves to protect your gums. Combined with mustard oil, this dynamic duo promotes comprehensive oral health.

Beets

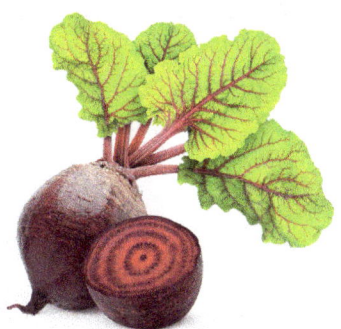

Unveiling the colorful secrets of beets - A Staining Sensation

Beware, the staining prowess of beets—a vegetable notorious for leaving its mark, even on your white tablecloth or favorite t-shirt. As with all staining foods, please exercise moderation when enjoying beets to safeguard against unexpected, unpleasant tooth discoloration.

Bell Peppers

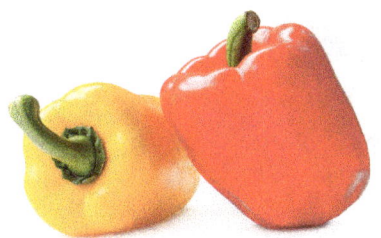

A Crunchy Ally for a Brighter Smile

Bell peppers are more than just a colorful addition to your plate—they're also a natural way to help whiten your teeth. Their crisp texture promotes saliva production, which helps wash away food particles and reduce plaque buildup.The high vitamin C content in bell peppers supports gum health and strengthens enamel, further contributing to a whiter smile. Enjoying bell peppers raw or adding them to your meals can naturally enhance your oral health and brighten your smile. Make these vibrant veggies a part of your diet and let your smile shine!

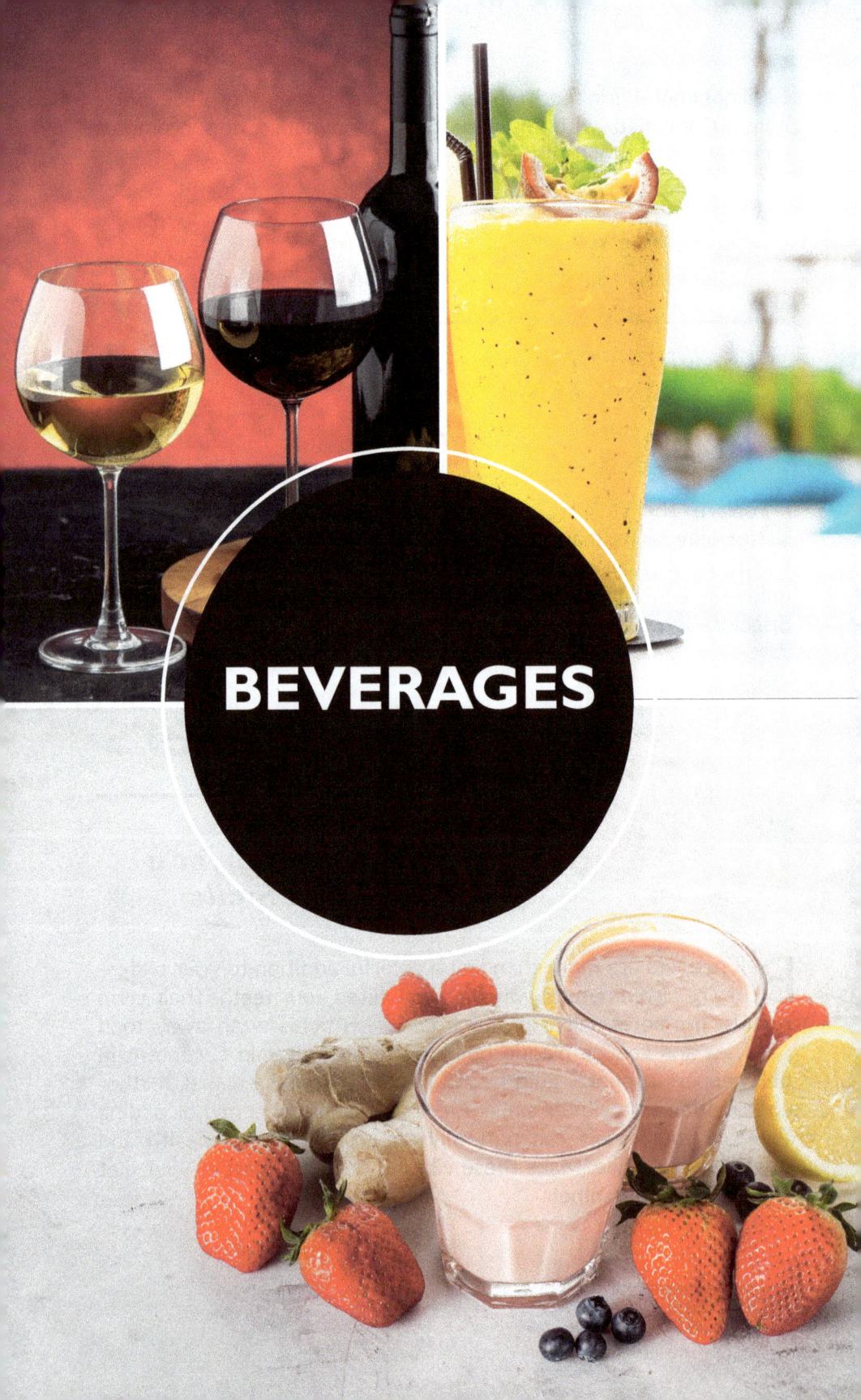

The Science of Seltzer Water

Because what's better than bubbles?

Seltzer water, or sparkling water, contains carbon dioxide (CO_2) which creates carbonic acid when dissolved in water. While this makes it slightly more acidic than regular water, its pH is still much lower than soft drinks or juices. However, acidity in general can weaken enamel over time, especially if consumed frequently throughout the day.

Key Points:

1. **Acidic Levels:** Seltzer water is mildly acidic
2. **No Added Sugars:** The great news is that plain seltzer doesn't contain sugars, which are the main culprits in tooth decay. So, no cavities from sugar here!
3. **Flavored Seltzers:** Be cautious with flavored varieties. Even without added sugar, the flavorings can sometimes increase acidity or may contain hidden sweeteners that are harmful to your teeth.

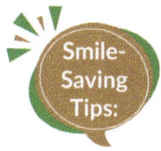

- **Moderation is Key:** Enjoy seltzer in moderation and try to pair it with meals, which naturally increase saliva flow and help neutralize acid.
- **Rinse with Water:** After drinking seltzer, rinse your mouth with plain water to wash away residual acid.
- **Avoid Brushing Right After** Don't brush immediately after having seltzer! Your enamel is slightly softened by the acidity, so give it some time to re-harden before brushing.

In summary, seltzer water in moderation is safe for your teeth, when followed up with a glass of plain water. This way, you can keep that smile bright while staying hydrated!

Sparkling Water

Friend or Foe to Your Smile?

Sparkling water, just like seltzer, is carbonated. This creates that fizzy sensation but also gives it mild acidity, which can affect your enamel over time.

What to Know:

1. **Acidity:** Sparkling water is more acidic than still water but far better for your teeth than soda or sugary drinks.

2. **Flavored Sparkling Waters:** Flavored varieties can sometimes have added citric acid, which increases the acidity, posing a greater risk to enamel. Also, watch out for brands sneaking in added sugars—sugar + acid is a bad combination for teeth.

3. **Tooth Erosion:** Drinking sparkling water alone isn't likely to cause significant enamel damage, but frequent, long-term consumption without proper care can contribute to enamel erosion, especially if it's flavored or consumed between meals.

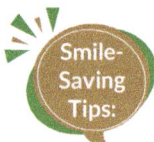

- **Stick to Plain:** If possible, stick to plain sparkling water without added flavors or sugars.

- **Pair with Food:** Drinking it with meals helps neutralize the acidity through saliva production, your mouth's natural defense mechanism.

- **Follow Up with Water:** Just like with seltzer, follow up with plain water to rinse any acid residue off your teeth.

Final Verdict:

Sparkling water, in moderation, isn't bad for your teeth, but be mindful of its acidity and potential flavor additives. The occasional bubbly drink is fine, balance is key to keeping your smile bright and healthy!

Club Soda

How It Impacts Your Teeth

Club soda is also carbonated like seltzer and sparkling water, but it's slightly different due to added minerals like sodium bicarbonate, sodium chloride, and potassium sulfate, which give it that distinctive taste.

The Dental Breakdown

1. Acidity: Like other carbonated drinks, club soda is mildly acidic and can contribute to enamel erosion over time if consumed frequently. The acid can wear down your enamel, making teeth more vulnerable to sensitivity and decay.

2. Added Minerals: The minerals in club soda (like sodium and potassium) don't necessarily harm teeth, but they also don't provide any added benefits to oral health. The focus is still on the acid content, not the minerals.

3. No Sugar: Just like plain sparkling water or seltzer, club soda usually doesn't contain sugar. Without sugar, there's no risk of feeding harmful bacteria in your mouth, which cause cavities.

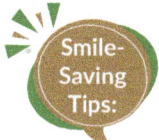
Smile-Saving Tips:

- **Moderation Is Key:** Enjoy club soda, but try not to make it your go-to drink throughout the day. Like other fizzy beverages, regular exposure to acid can slowly wear away enamel.

- **Watch Out for Flavor Additions:** If your club soda has added flavors, check the label for hidden sugars or acids (like citric acid), which could make it harmful to your teeth.

- **Rinse with Water:** Follow up your club soda with a sip of still water to wash away residual acid and keep your enamel safe.

- **Wait Before Brushing:** If you've been sipping club soda, give your teeth about 30 minutes before brushing to allow the enamel to reharden.

Verdict:

Club soda isn't inherently bad for your teeth, but like any acidic drink, it can weaken enamel over time with frequent consumption. It's best to enjoy it in moderation, and always give your teeth a little TLC afterward with a quick rinse of plain water!

Tonic Water

A Trickier Drink for Your Smile

Tonic water is carbonated, just like other fizzy drinks, but the key difference is it contains quinine for that signature bitter taste, along with added sugars. This combination makes it potentially more harmful to your teeth compared to plain sparkling water or club soda.

Why Tonic Water Can Be Bad for Your Teeth:

1. Sugar Content: The biggest issue with tonic water is the sugar. Most tonic waters contain a significant amount of sugar (similar to soft drinks), and sugar is one of the top culprits of tooth decay. When sugars mix with the bacteria in your mouth, they create acids that can erode enamel and lead to cavities.

2. Acidity: Tonic water is also acidic. The acidity, combined with sugar, forms a one-two punch that can soften enamel, making it easier for cavities to form, and causing long-term enamel wear.

3. Quinine: While quinine itself isn't harmful to your teeth, it doesn't do anything to mitigate the sugar and acid content. It's primarily the sugars and acids that do the damage.

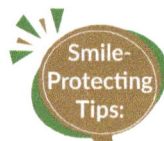

Smile-Protecting Tips:

- **Limit Frequency:** If you enjoy tonic water (especially in cocktails), try to limit how often you drink it. Frequent exposure to sugar and acid puts your enamel at greater risk.

- **Rinse After Drinking:** After enjoying tonic water, rinse your mouth with plain water to help wash away the sugars and acids. This will help protect your enamel from further damage.

- **Drink with Meals:** If possible, drink tonic water during meals when your saliva production increases, which helps neutralize acids and protect your enamel.

Verdict Decision:

Tonic water is more harmful to your teeth than plain sparkling water or club soda due to its high sugar content and acidity. If you're trying to keep your smile bright and cavity-free, it's best to enjoy tonic water occasionally rather than regularly.

Energy Drinks

High-Energy, High-Risk for Your Teeth

Energy drinks are loaded with sugar and have high acidity levels, making them one of the worst beverages for your teeth. They promise a quick boost in energy, but they come with long-term consequences for your smile.

Why Energy Drinks Are Bad for Your Teeth:

1. High Sugar Content: Most energy drinks are packed with sugar—sometimes even more than sodas. The sugar feeds harmful bacteria in your mouth, which then produce acids that erode your enamel and lead to cavities.

2. Low pH Levels (High Acidity): The acidity of energy drinks is particularly concerning, with pH levels often below 3. This means they are highly acidic, which weakens enamel almost immediately upon contact. Once enamel is eroded, it can't regenerate, leaving your teeth vulnerable to decay and sensitivity.

3. Frequent Consumption: People often sip energy drinks throughout the day, keeping their teeth in a prolonged acid bath. This constant exposure prevents saliva from doing its job of neutralizing acids and protecting teeth.

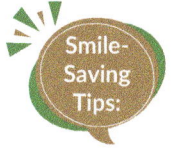
Smile-Saving Tips:

- **Limit Your Intake:** Reduce how often you drink energy drinks to minimize the harm to your teeth.
- **Choose Sugar-Free Options:** While sugar-free energy drinks still have high acidity, cutting out the sugar helps reduce the risk of cavities.
- **Rinse with Water:** After consuming an energy drink, rinse your mouth with water to wash away the acids.
- **Wait Before Brushing:** Avoid brushing your teeth right after drinking energy drinks. The acidity temporarily softens enamel, so wait at least 30 minutes before brushing to give your enamel time to re-harden.

The Last Word:

Energy drinks are one of the worst culprits when it comes to damaging teeth. Between their high sugar content and acidity, they can cause significant enamel erosion, tooth decay, and sensitivity if consumed regularly. If you need a boost of energy, try to reach for healthier alternatives like water, unsweetened tea, or black coffee.

Sports Drinks

Hydrating Your Body, Hurting Your Teeth

While sports drinks help replenish electrolytes after physical activity, they come with a hidden downside: high sugar content and acidity. Both of these factors can wreak havoc on your teeth, especially with regular consumption.

Why Sports Drinks Are Bad for Your Teeth:

1. **High Sugar Content:** Most sports drinks are loaded with sugar, which contributes to tooth decay. The sugar interacts with the bacteria in your mouth, creating acids that attack tooth enamel. This leads to cavities, especially when you're sipping on these drinks throughout the day or after workouts.

2. **Acidic pH Levels:** The pH level of sports drinks ranges from 3 to 4, making them quite acidic. This acidity can soften and erode enamel over time, leading to sensitive teeth and increased vulnerability to decay.

3. **Frequent Sipping:** Many people sip on sports drinks during and after workouts, keeping their teeth in prolonged contact with sugar and acid. With saliva levels often reduced during physical activity, your mouth loses one of its best defenses against acid, leaving teeth more susceptible to damage.

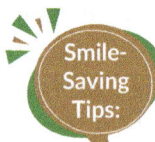
Smile-Saving Tips:

- **Opt for Water:** For most people, water is all you need to rehydrate after exercise. It's the safest option for your teeth and your health.
- **Limit Sports Drinks to Intense Workouts:** If you're doing endurance training or intense exercise, sports drinks can be helpful but try to limit them to these occasions.
- **Rinse with Water:** After consuming a sports drink, rinse your mouth with water to wash away the sugar and acid.
- **Avoid Brushing Immediately:** Wait at least 30 minutes before brushing your teeth after drinking sports drinks to allow your enamel to reharden.

Final Determination:

Sports drinks are acidic and sugary, which makes them bad news for your teeth. They can lead to enamel erosion, cavities, and sensitivity, especially if consumed frequently. Whenever possible, reach for water to keep your body hydrated and your teeth healthy.

Alcoholic Beverages

Not So Friendly to Your Teeth

Alcoholic beverages are a sneaky culprit when it comes to oral health. While you might think of them as part of a night out or a relaxing evening, many of these drinks can be quite harmful to your teeth. Here's what to know about alcoholic beverages.

Alcohol can be acidic, drying, and often paired with sugary mixers, making it a triple threat to your oral health. Let's explore the main ways alcohol can damage your teeth.

Why Alcoholic Beverages Are Bad for Your Teeth:

1. **High Acidity:** Many alcoholic beverages—especially wine, beer, and cocktails—are acidic. Drinks like wine (especially white) and beer have low pH levels, which can weaken and erode tooth enamel over time, making teeth more prone to decay and sensitivity.

2. **Sugar Content:** Cocktails and mixed drinks are often loaded with sugar, from syrups, fruit juices, and soda. Sugar is a major cause of tooth decay because it feeds bacteria in your mouth that produce enamel-eroding acids.

3. **Dehydration and Dry Mouth:** Alcohol causes dry mouth by reducing saliva production. Saliva is your mouth's natural defense against acids and bacteria, and a lack of it can lead to enamel erosion, tooth decay, and bad breath.

4. **Staining:** Drinks like red wine and dark liquors are notorious for staining teeth. They contain pigments and tannins that cling to the enamel, leading to discoloration and dullness over time.

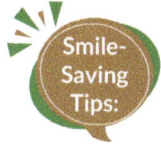
Smile-Saving Tips:

- **Alternate with Water:** Drink water in between alcoholic beverages to rinse your mouth and keep hydrated. This helps wash away acids and sugars and stimulates saliva production.

- **Avoid Sugary Mixers:** Stick to mixers like soda water or tonic water (in moderation) instead of sugary sodas or juices in your cocktails.
- **Limit Staining Drinks:** Be mindful of how often you drink red wine or dark liquors, and consider drinking them through a straw to reduce contact with your teeth.
- **Rinse with Water Post-Drink:** After enjoying alcohol, rinse your mouth with water to remove sugars and acids.
- **Wait Before Brushing:** Since alcohol softens enamel, wait at least 30 minutes after drinking before brushing your teeth to avoid further damage to softened enamel.

Last Call:

Alcoholic beverages can be tough on your teeth due to their acidity, sugar content, and drying effects. Over time, they can lead to enamel erosion, cavities, and stains. While it's fine to enjoy alcohol in moderation, being mindful of its impact on your oral health and taking steps to protect your teeth can help maintain a bright, healthy smile.

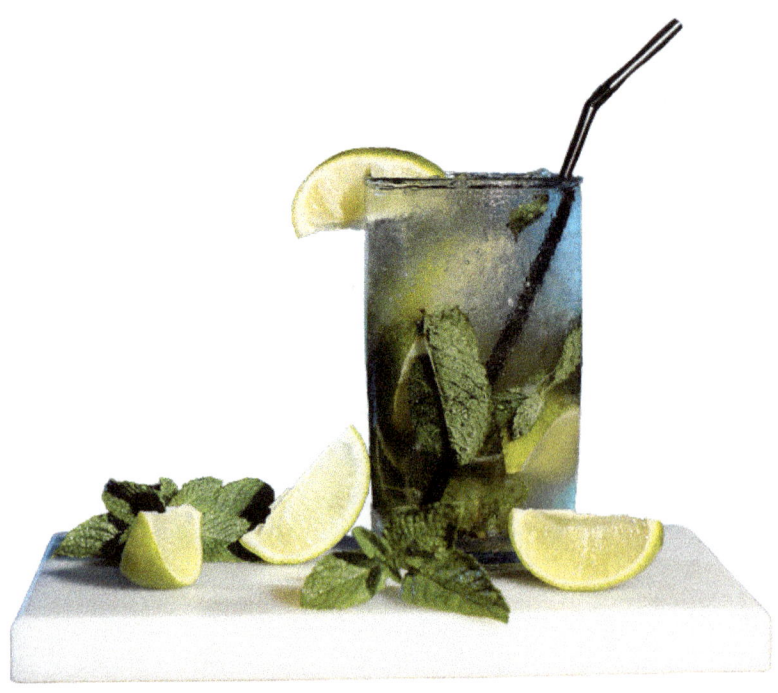

Coffee

Energizing, but Tough on Your Teeth

While coffee might kickstart your day, there are often some unintended side effects for your smile. Whether you drink it black or with added cream and sugar, coffee has some negative qualities that can be harmful to your teeth.

Why Coffee Can Be Bad for Your Teeth:

1. **Staining:** Due to its dark pigments, coffee is notorious for staining teeth. These pigments (called tannins) can stick to the enamel and over time lead to yellow or brown discoloration, dulling the brightness of your smile.

2. **Acidity:** Coffee is slightly acidic, with a pH around 5. While not as acidic as some other beverages, regular consumption can still weaken enamel, especially when consumed throughout the day. Once enamel is eroded, teeth can become more sensitive and prone to decay.

3. **Added Sugars and Creamers:** Many people enjoy coffee with sugar, flavored syrups, or creamers, which can turn a simple cup of coffee into a cavity risk. The added sugars feed harmful bacteria in the mouth, creating acids that contribute to tooth decay.

4. **Dry Mouth:** Coffee, like alcohol, is a diuretic, meaning it can dry out your mouth. Reduced saliva flow makes it harder for your mouth to wash away acids and bacteria, increasing the risk of cavities and bad breath.

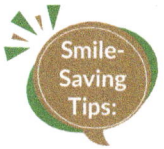

- **Drink in One Sitting:** Instead of sipping on coffee throughout the day, drink it in a shorter time period to minimize prolonged exposure to acids and staining agents.

- **Rinse with Water:** After enjoying your coffee, rinse your mouth with water to wash away acids and pigments before they can settle on your teeth.

- **Limit Sugary Additives:** Try to avoid adding sugar or sweetened creamers to your coffee. If you need a sweetener, consider sugarfree options.
- **Wait Before Brushing:** Don't brush your teeth immediately after drinking coffee, as brushing can soften your enamel. Wait about 30 minutes to give your enamel time to harden.

End Result:

While coffee itself isn't the worst offender, it can lead to staining, enamel erosion, and increased cavity risk, especially if consumed with sugar. With a few simple habits—like rinsing with water and drinking in moderation—you can still enjoy your daily cup of joe while keeping your teeth bright and healthy.

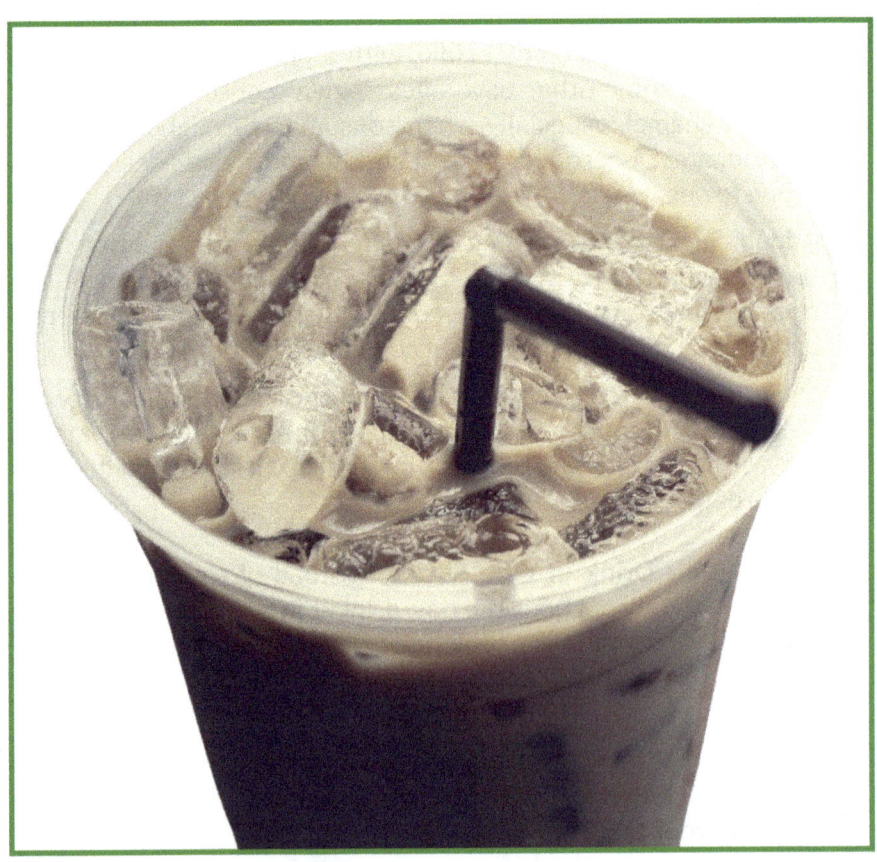

Tea

A Steeped Debate for Your Teeth

Tea is a bit of a mixed bag when it comes to oral health. Here's a comprehensive look at how tea impacts your teeth.

Tea is often touted for its health benefits, but its effects on your teeth can vary depending on the type and how it's consumed. Let's explore the pros and cons:

Why Tea Can Be Bad for Your Teeth:

1. **Staining:** Both black and green teas contain tannins, which can cause staining. Black tea is particularly notorious for this, as it can lead to yellow or brown discoloration on teeth. Even green tea, though lighter, can contribute to some degree of staining.

2. **Acidity:** Tea has a relatively low pH, making it slightly acidic. While not as acidic as soda or citrus juices, the acidity in tea can gradually weaken enamel, especially if consumed frequently.

3. **Added Sugars:** If you add sugar or honey to your tea, you're introducing a cavity risk. Sugars feed bacteria that produce acids, which contribute to tooth decay and enamel erosion.

4. **Dry Mouth:** Tea, especially caffeinated varieties, can have a mild diuretic effect, potentially leading to dry mouth. Saliva is crucial for neutralizing acids and protecting enamel, so reduced saliva flow can increase the risk of tooth decay.

Why Tea Can Be Good for Your Teeth:

1. **Fluoride Content:** Many teas, particularly black tea, contain fluoride, which can help strengthen enamel and protect against cavities. However, the fluoride content is generally not high enough to replace good oral hygiene practices.

2. **Antioxidants:** Tea, especially green tea, is rich in antioxidants that can benefit overall health, including oral health. Green tea contains polyphenols that have antimicrobial properties and may help reduce bacteria in the mouth.

3. **Less Sugar:** Unsweetened tea is a better choice for your teeth compared to sugary beverages. It's less likely to contribute to cavities and doesn't have the high sugar content that exacerbates tooth decay.

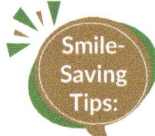

- **Opt for Unsweetened Tea:** To avoid the added sugar risks, drink tea without sugar or sweeteners.
- **Rinse Your Mouth:** After drinking tea, especially if it's a dark variety, rinse your mouth with water to help reduce staining and wash away acids.
- **Drink Water:** Balance tea consumption with plenty of water to stay hydrated and stimulate saliva flow.
- **Regular Oral Hygiene:** Maintain a consistent brushing and flossing routine to combat staining and protect enamel.

Final Assessment:

Tea can be both beneficial and detrimental to your teeth. While it offers some health benefits and is less harmful than sugary drinks, its potential for staining, acidity, and dry mouth means it's important to enjoy it in moderation and follow good oral care practices.

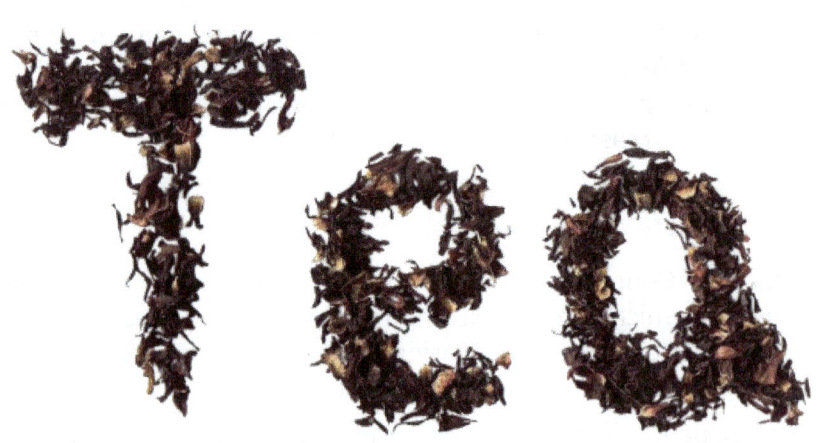

Regular Iced Tea

Harmful but Less

Why It's Bad for Your Teeth:

1. Staining: Regular iced tea, especially black tea, contains tannins that can cause staining over time. These tannins cling to tooth enamel, leading to discoloration.
2. Acidity: Iced tea is acidic, with a pH ranging from about 4 to 3.
3. While not as acidic as sodas or citrus juices, the acidity can still contribute to enamel erosion, particularly with frequent consumption.

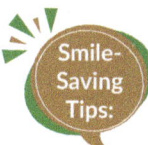

- **Rinse with Water:** After drinking iced tea, rinse your mouth with water to help neutralize acids and wash away tannins.
- **Use a Straw:** When possible, use a straw to reduce direct contact with your teeth.
- **Limit Consumption:** Enjoy iced tea in moderation to minimize staining and acid exposure.
- **Maintain Oral Hygiene:** Brush and floss regularly to help combat staining and maintain healthy enamel.

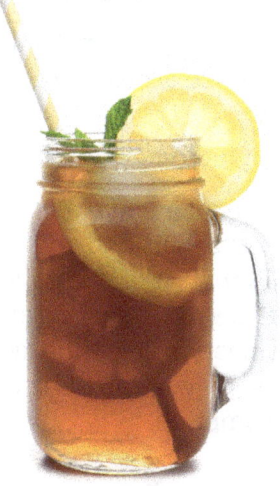

Sweetened Iced Tea

Greater Risks

Why It's Worse for Your Teeth:

1. **High Sugar Content:** Sweetened iced tea contains added sugars that feed harmful bacteria in the mouth. This leads to acid production that erodes enamel and increases the risk of cavities.
2. **Staining:** Like regular iced tea, sweetened iced tea can still cause staining due to tannins.
3. **Acidity:** Sweetened iced tea retains the acidity of regular iced tea, which can contribute to enamel erosion.

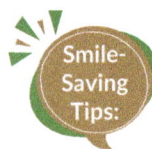

Smile-Saving Tips:

- **Opt for Unsweetened:** Choose unsweetened iced tea or reduce the amount of sugar added to cut down on cavity risk.
- **Rinse with Water:** After consuming sweetened iced tea, rinse your mouth with water to help wash away sugars and acids.
- **Brush After 30 Minutes:** Avoid brushing your teeth immediately after drinking to prevent damage to softened enamel. Wait about 30 minutes to brush.
- **Monitor Intake:** Limit the consumption of sweetened iced tea to reduce exposure to sugars and acids.

Final Outcome:

Both regular and sweetened iced tea can be harmful to your teeth due to their acidity and potential for staining. Sweetened iced tea presents additional risks due to its high sugar content, which can exacerbate tooth decay. By making a few adjustments—like opting for unsweetened versions, rinsing your mouth with water, and maintaining good oral hygiene—you can mitigate some of the risks associated with iced tea consumption.

Red vs. White Wine

How They Affect Your Teeth

Why It's Bad for Your Teeth:

1. **Staining:** Red wine is infamous for its ability to stain teeth. The deep pigments (anthocyanins and tannins) in red wine can cling to enamel and lead to discoloration over time.
2. **Acidity:** Red wine is acidic (pH around 3-4), which can erode enamel. The combination of acidity and staining pigments makes red wine particularly harmful to tooth color and health.

Why It's Bad for Your Teeth:

1. **Acidity:** White wine is also acidic (pH around 3), which can weaken enamel and increase the risk of decay and sensitivity. The acidity in white wine can soften enamel and make it more susceptible to erosion.
2. **Staining Potential:** Although less staining than red wine, white wine can still contribute to enamel erosion, which can make teeth more prone to discoloration from other sources.

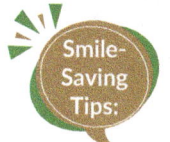

General Tips for Both Red and White Wine:

1. **Rinse with Water:** After drinking wine, rinse your mouth with water to help wash away acids and pigments. This can reduce the risk of enamel erosion and staining.
2. **Drink Water Between Glasses:** Alternating wine with water can help dilute the acidity and reduce the impact on your teeth.
3. **Use a Straw:** While not always practical with wine, using a straw can minimize contact with your teeth, especially for white wine.
4. **Brush Teeth Wisely:** Wait at least 30 minutes after drinking wine before brushing your teeth. Brushing immediately after can damage softened enamel.

5. **Regular Oral Care:** Maintain a robust oral hygiene routine with regular brushing and flossing. Consider using a whitening toothpaste to help manage discoloration and maintain oral health.
6. **Consider Dental Products:** Use fluoride treatments or remineralizing toothpaste to strengthen enamel and protect against acidity.

Differences Between Red and White Wine:

- Acidity: Both red and white wines are acidic, but white wines are often more acidic than red wines. This higher acidity in white wines
- can more readily soften enamel.
- Staining: Red wine has a higher staining potential due to its darker pigments and tannins. White wine is less likely to stain but can still contribute to enamel erosion.

Final Say:

Both red and white wines can be detrimental to your teeth, albeit in different ways. Red wine is more likely to cause staining, while white wine's higher acidity poses a risk for enamel erosion. By taking steps to minimize contact and protect your teeth, you can enjoy wine in moderation while preserving your smile.

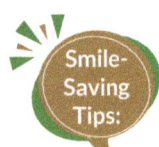

- Rinse with water after a glass of wine to wash away acids and tannins.
- Pair wine with cheese or other foods that help neutralize acid.
- Avoid brushing your teeth immediately after drinking—wait 30 minutes.

More on Wine in the "W" Section.

Fruit Juices

The Sweet and Sour Impact on Your Teeth

Fruit juices, especially when consumed in excess, can pose significant risks to your oral health. Their natural sugars and acidity can be particularly problematic.

Why Fruit Juices Can Be Bad for Your Teeth:

1. **High Sugar Content:** Fruit juices, even those labeled as 100% fruit juice, contain high levels of natural sugars. These sugars feed bacteria in your mouth, leading to acid production that erodes enamel and increases the risk of cavities.

2. **Acidity:** Many fruit juices, such as orange juice, grapefruit juice, and apple juice, are highly acidic. The acidity can weaken enamel, making teeth more susceptible to decay and sensitivity. Frequent exposure to acidic beverages can accelerate enamel erosion.

3. **Frequent Consumption:** Drinking fruit juice throughout the day prolongs the exposure of your teeth to sugars and acids. This extended contact can exacerbate enamel erosion and increase the risk of tooth decay.

4. **Potential for Staining:** Some fruit juices, particularly those with dark pigments like grape juice, can contribute to staining and discoloration of teeth over time.

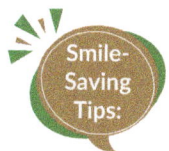

Smile-Saving Tips:

- **Opt for Water:** Whenever possible, choose water over fruit juice to avoid the high sugar and acid content. Water is the best choice for maintaining overall oral health and hydration.
- **Limit Juice Intake:** If you do consume fruit juice, do so in moderation. Try to limit it to mealtimes rather than sipping it throughout the day.
- **Choose 100% Fruit Juice:** If you choose to drink fruit juice, select 100% fruit juice with no added sugars. Even then, it's best to consume it in small amounts.

- **Dilute Juice with Water:** Diluting fruit juice with water can reduce its sugar and acidity levels, making it less harmful to your teeth.
- **Rinse with Water:** After drinking fruit juice, rinse your mouth with water to help wash away sugars and acids.
- **Wait Before Brushing:** Avoid brushing your teeth immediately after consuming fruit juice. The acidity can soften enamel, and brushing right away can cause additional damage. Wait at least 30 minutes before brushing.

Last Judgement:

Fruit juices can be detrimental to your dental health due to their high sugar content and acidity. They can contribute to enamel erosion, tooth decay, and staining. By limiting intake, diluting juices, and following good oral hygiene practices, you can enjoy fruit juice while minimizing its impact on your teeth.

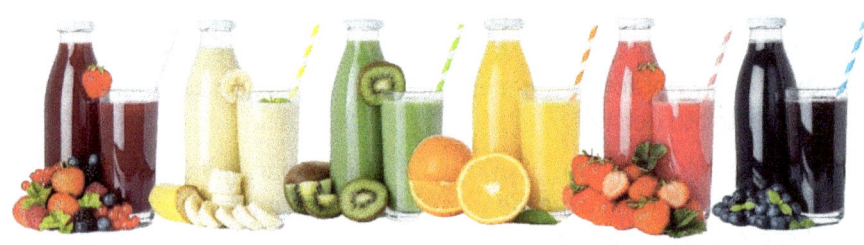

Cola and Diet Cola

How They Affect Your Teeth

Cola

Why It's Bad for Your Teeth:

1. **High Sugar Content:** Regular cola contains high levels of sugar, which feeds harmful bacteria in your mouth. These bacteria produce acids that erode enamel and increase the risk of cavities.
2. **High Acidity:** Cola is highly acidic, with a pH around 2.5. This acidity can weaken and erode tooth enamel, leading to increased sensitivity and decay over time.
3. **Staining:** The dark pigments in cola can cause staining and discoloration of teeth. Frequent consumption can lead to noticeable dark spots or yellowing.

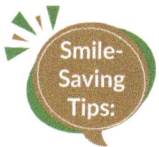

- **Drink in Moderation:** Limit your intake of regular cola to reduce exposure to sugar and acids.
- **Rinse with Water:** After drinking cola, rinse your mouth with water to help neutralize acids and wash away sugar.
- **Use a Straw:** When drinking cola, use a straw to minimize contact with your teeth.
- **Wait to Brush:** Avoid brushing your teeth immediately after drinking cola. The acidity can soften enamel, and brushing right away can cause additional damage. Wait about 30 minutes before brushing.

Diet Cola

Why It's Bad for Your Teeth:

1. Acidity: Diet cola is also highly acidic, with a pH similar to that of regular cola. This acidity can erode enamel, making teeth more susceptible to decay and sensitivity.
2. Staining: Like regular cola, diet cola contains dark pigments that can contribute to staining and discoloration of teeth.
3. No Sugar, But Still Harmful: While diet cola contains artificial sweeteners instead of sugar, the high acidity remains a concern. The absence of sugar doesn't eliminate the risk of enamel erosion and staining.

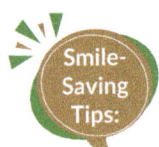

- **Limit Consumption:** Even though diet cola has no sugar, its acidity can still damage enamel, so it's best to consume it in moderation.
- **Rinse with Water:** Rinse your mouth with water after drinking diet cola to help neutralize the acids.
- **Use a Straw:** Use a straw to reduce the direct contact of the acidic beverage with your teeth.
- **Wait Before Brushing:** As with regular cola, wait at least 30 minutes before brushing your teeth to prevent damaging softened enamel.

Final Say:

Both cola and diet cola can negatively impact your dental health. Regular cola is harmful due to its high sugar content and acidity, while diet cola, though sugar-free, remains acidic and can still lead to enamel erosion and staining. By limiting your consumption and following good oral hygiene practices, you can help mitigate these risks.

Flavored Water & Vitamin Waters

Impact on Your Teeth

Flavored Water

Why It Can Be Bad for Your Teeth:

1. **Acidity:** Many flavored waters contain added acids, such as citric acid, to enhance their taste. This acidity can erode enamel, making teeth more susceptible to decay and sensitivity.
2. **Added Sugars or Sweeteners:** Some flavored waters contain added sugars or artificial sweeteners. Even if the sugar content is low, the acids can still contribute to enamel erosion.

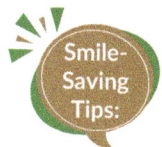

- **Check Labels:** Look for flavored waters with no added sugars or artificial sweeteners. Opt for those with minimal acidity.
- **Rinse with Water:** After drinking flavored water, rinse your mouth with plain water to help neutralize acids and wash away any residual flavoring.
- **Drink Plain Water:** Whenever possible, choose plain water over flavored options to avoid potential acidity and sugar issues.

Vitamin Waters

Why They Can Be Bad for Your Teeth:

1. **High Sugar Content:** Many vitamin waters contain added sugars to improve flavor. These sugars can contribute to tooth decay by feeding harmful bacteria in the mouth.
2. **Acidity:** Vitamin waters often contain citric acid and other acidic ingredients. The acidity can weaken enamel, leading to increased risk of decay and sensitivity.

3. **Staining:** Some vitamin waters have artificial colors that can lead to staining and discoloration of teeth.

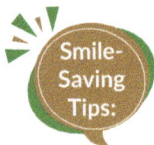

Smile-Saving Tips:

- **Choose Low-Sugar Options:** Opt for vitamin waters with low or no added sugars. Check the label for sugar content and artificial sweeteners.
- **Rinse with Water:** After drinking vitamin water, rinse your mouth with plain water to help neutralize acids and wash away sugars.
- **Limit Intake:** Consume vitamin waters in moderation. Regular consumption can increase the risk of enamel erosion and decay.

Final Outcome:

Both flavored waters and vitamin waters can have negative effects on your dental health due to their acidity and, in some cases, added sugars. Flavored waters can erode enamel if they contain acids, while vitamin waters pose additional risks with high sugar content and acidity. By opting for low-acid and low-sugar options and maintaining good oral hygiene practices, you can minimize the impact on your teeth.

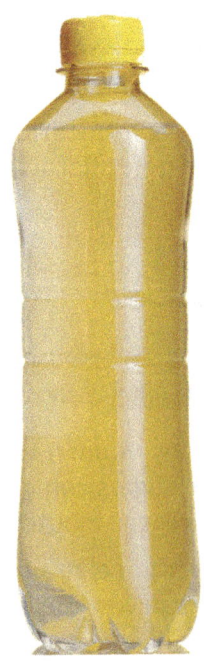

Milkshakes and Smoothies

Impact on Your Teeth

Milkshakes

Why They Can Be Bad for Your Teeth:

1. **High Sugar Content:** Milkshakes are typically high in sugars due to the ice cream or syrup used to flavor them. The sugars can feed harmful bacteria in your mouth, leading to tooth decay and cavities.

2. **Acidity:** Some milkshakes contain acidic ingredients, like certain fruits or flavorings, which can contribute to enamel erosion over time.

3. **Sticky Texture:** Milkshakes can have a thick, sticky texture that might cling to your teeth, making it harder for saliva to wash away sugars and acids.

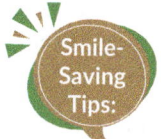

Smile-Saving Tips:

- **Moderate Consumption:** Enjoy milkshakes occasionally rather than as a regular treat to limit sugar exposure.
- **Rinse with Water:** After drinking a milkshake, rinse your mouth with water to help remove sugars and acids.
- **Choose Lower-Sugar Options:** Opt for milkshakes made with less sugar or substitute with lower-sugar ice cream or frozen yogurt.

Smoothies

Why They Can Be Bad for Your Teeth:

1. **High Sugar Content:** Smoothies, especially those made with sweetened yogurt, honey, or fruit juices, can be high in natural sugars. These sugars can promote tooth decay if consumed frequently.
2. **Acidity:** Many smoothies contain acidic fruits like oranges, pineapples, and berries. The acidity can erode enamel, making teeth more vulnerable to decay.
3. **Potential for Staining:** Smoothies made with dark berries or other pigmented ingredients can contribute to staining and discoloration of teeth.

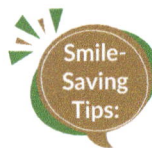

Smile-Saving Tips:

- **Use Low-Sugar Ingredients:** Make smoothies with low-sugar or unsweetened yogurt and avoid adding extra sugars. Opt for fresh or frozen fruits rather than fruit juices.
- **Balance with Water:** Add a good amount of water or unsweetened almond milk to your smoothie to reduce the concentration of sugars and acids.
- **Rinse with Water:** After drinking a smoothie, rinse your mouth with water to help dilute and wash away sugars and acids.
- **Incorporate Teeth-Friendly Ingredients:** Consider adding ingredients that are beneficial for oral health, such as leafy greens, which can help balance acidity.

Last Judgement:

Both milkshakes and smoothies can pose risks to dental health due to their sugar content and potential acidity. Milkshakes are particularly high in sugar and can be sticky, while smoothies can have high sugar content and acidity, depending on their ingredients. By consuming these beverages in moderation, opting for lower-sugar versions, and following good oral hygiene practices, you can enjoy them while minimizing their impact on your teeth.

Blackberries

A Sweet Way to a Brighter Smile

Blackberries are not just delicious—they can also help whiten your teeth naturally. Packed with antioxidants and vitamins, blackberries support overall oral health by reducing plaque buildup and preventing gum inflammation. Their high fiber content stimulates saliva production, which helps cleanse your teeth and remove surface stains. Additionally, blackberries contain natural acids that can gently break down discoloration. Incorporating these juicy berries into your diet can contribute to a whiter, healthier smile while enjoying their sweet taste. Add blackberries to your daily routine and savor the benefits of a naturally radiant smile!

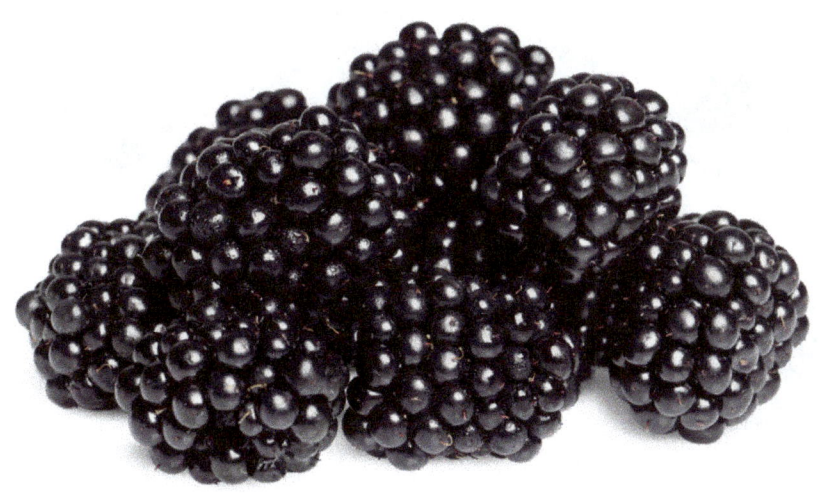

Blueberries

A Berry Good Choice for a Whiter Smile

Blueberries are more than just a tasty treat—they can also help whiten your teeth naturally. Rich in antioxidants and vitamins, blueberries promote oral health by reducing plaque and supporting gum health. Their high fiber content encourages saliva production, which helps to wash away food particles and bacteria that can cause staining. Additionally, blueberries contain natural compounds that can gently lift surface stains from your teeth. Including blueberries in your diet is a delicious way to enhance your oral care routine and achieve a brighter, healthier smile. Enjoy these vibrant berries and let your smile shine!

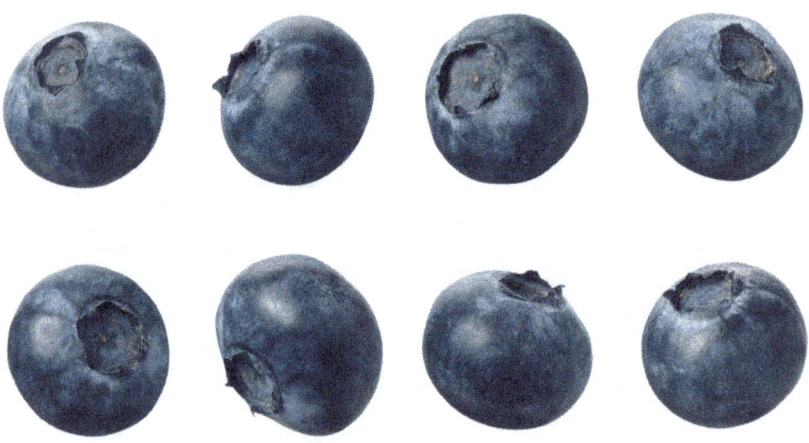

Bok Choy

A Crisp Choice for a Brighter Smile

Bok choy isn't just a crunchy, nutrient-packed vegetable—it also helps naturally whiten your teeth. Its high water content and crisp texture stimulate saliva production, which aids in washing away food particles and reducing plaque buildup. The calcium and vitamins found in bok choy contribute to strong enamel and overall oral health, further supporting a whiter smile. Incorporate bok choy into your meals to enjoy its benefits for a naturally brighter, healthier smile while adding a delightful crunch to your diet.

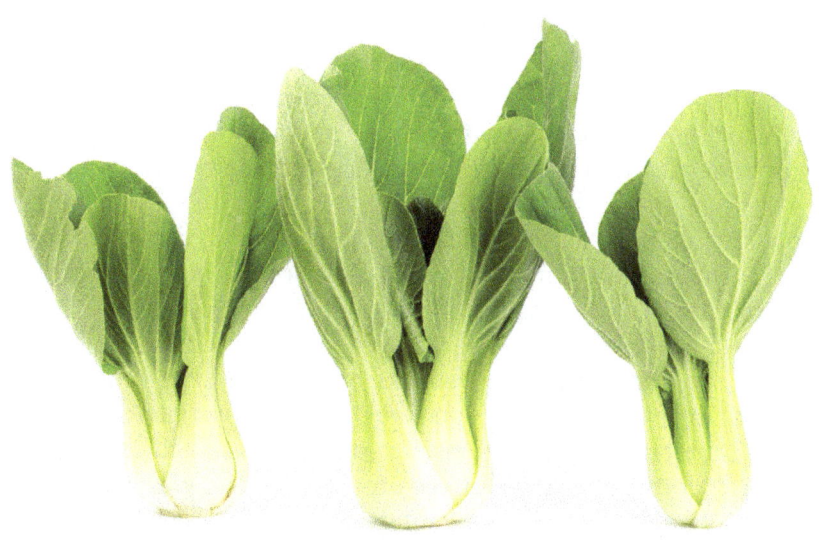

Broccoli

Embrace the Crunchy Goodness

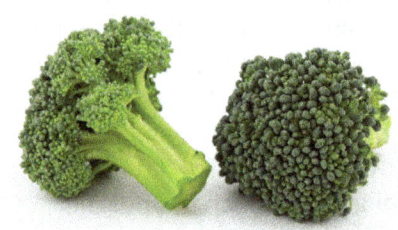

Broccoli, already celebrated as a "miracle food" for its rich content of vitamins, fiber, and calcium, might also be a powerhouse for oral health. A study published in the European Journal of Dentistry in by Brazilian researchers found that broccoli could be a top contender for tooth protection, thanks to its high iron content.

The study focused on enamel erosion, which not only dulls teeth but also increases the risk of cavities and decay. Remarkably, when teeth were exposed to broccoli extract before soda, there was less enamel erosion. Researchers believe that iron may form a protective coating on teeth, shielding them from enamel-eroding acids. If broccoli isn't your favorite, other iron-rich foods like spinach or liver might offer similar benefits when eaten before acidic drinks or meals.

Instead of steaming, enjoy the crisp texture of this green vegetable in its raw form. As you munch away, let the broccoli's high fiber content scrub your teeth, providing a quick and natural mid-day brush.

Furthermore, the nutritional benefits of broccoli extend beyond its toothcleaning properties. Its high levels of iron can coat your enamel, offering protection against stains, harmful bacteria, and acid erosion. Incorporate broccoli into your diet for a delicious way to promote dental health and maintain a radiant smile.

If broccoli isn't your favorite, other iron-rich foods like spinach or liver might offer similar benefits when eaten before acidic drinks or meals.

Brussels Sprouts

A Nutritious Boost for a Brighter Smile

Brussels sprouts are not only a nutrient-rich vegetable but also a natural ally for whitening your teeth. Their high fiber content promotes saliva production, which helps cleanse your teeth and reduce plaque buildup. Additionally, Brussels sprouts are packed with vitamins and minerals, including vitamin C and calcium, which strengthen enamel and support overall oral health. Incorporating these tiny powerhouses into your diet can contribute to a naturally whiter smile while providing essential nutrients for your body. Enjoy Brussels sprouts as a delicious side dish and let your smile benefit from their natural tooth-whitening properties!

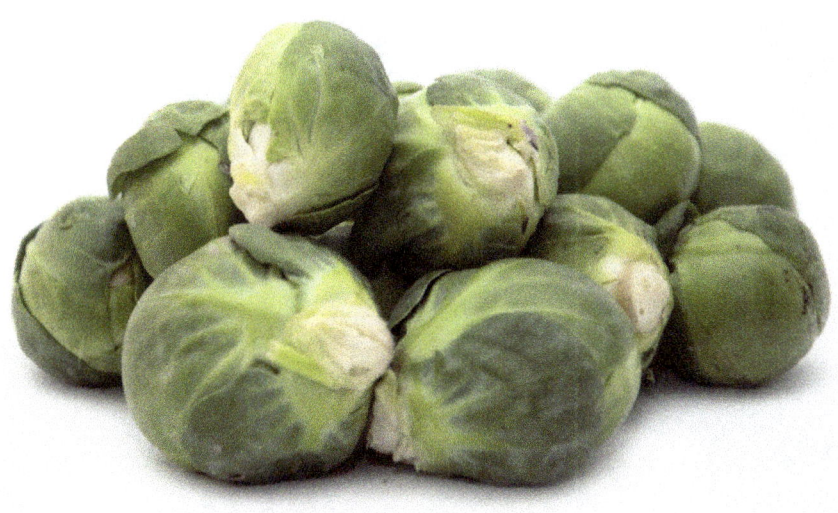

C

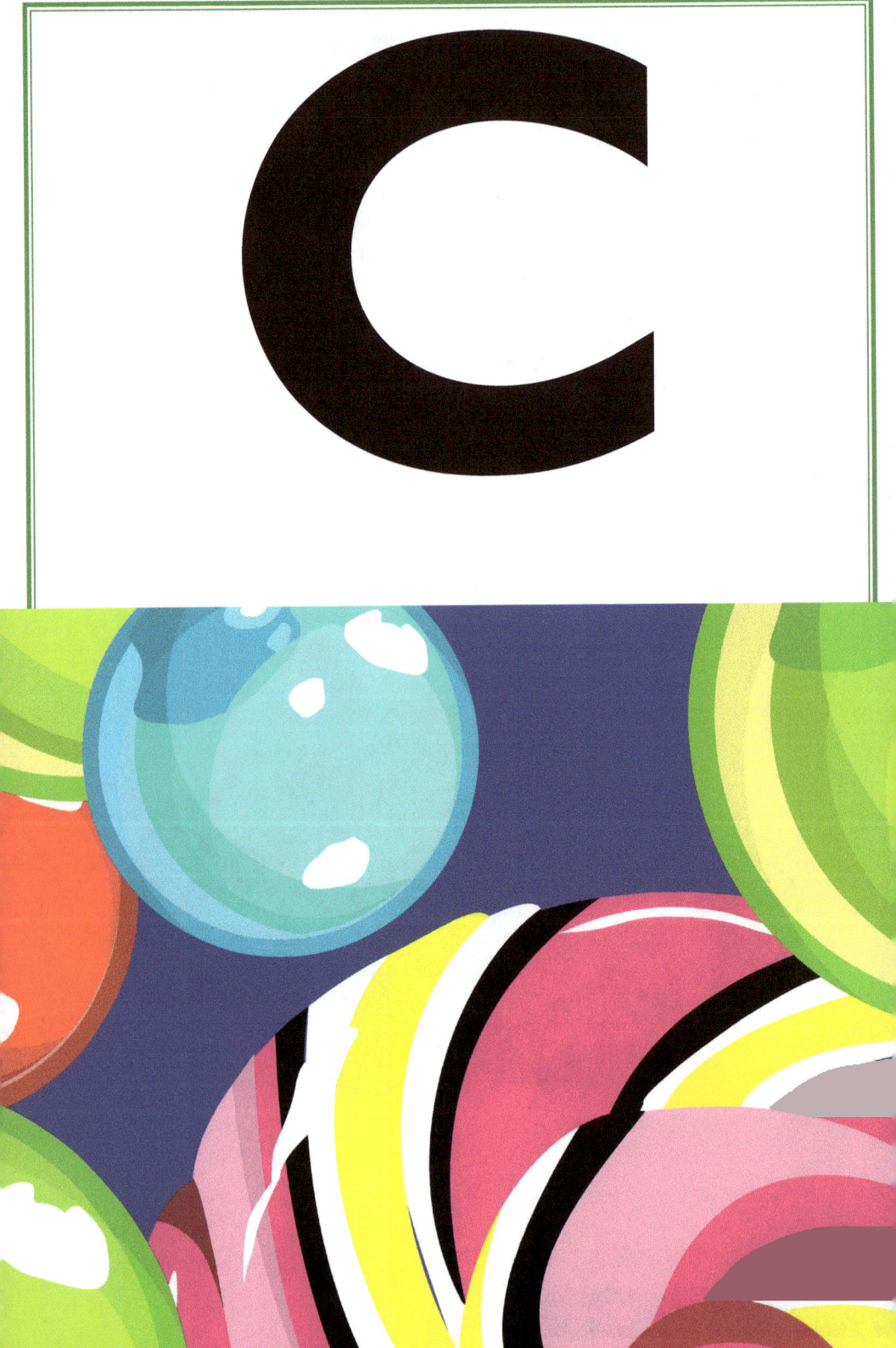

Cabbage

A Crunchy Helper for a Brighter Smile

Cabbage is more than just a versatile vegetable—it can also support a naturally whiter smile. Its crunchy texture helps stimulate saliva production, which is crucial for washing away food particles and reducing plaque buildup. Additionally, cabbage is rich in vitamins and minerals, including vitamin C, which supports gum health and strengthens enamel. By incorporating cabbage into your meals, you can enjoy its natural toothcleansing benefits while contributing to a brighter, healthier smile. Add this leafy green to your diet and let its natural properties enhance your oral care routine!

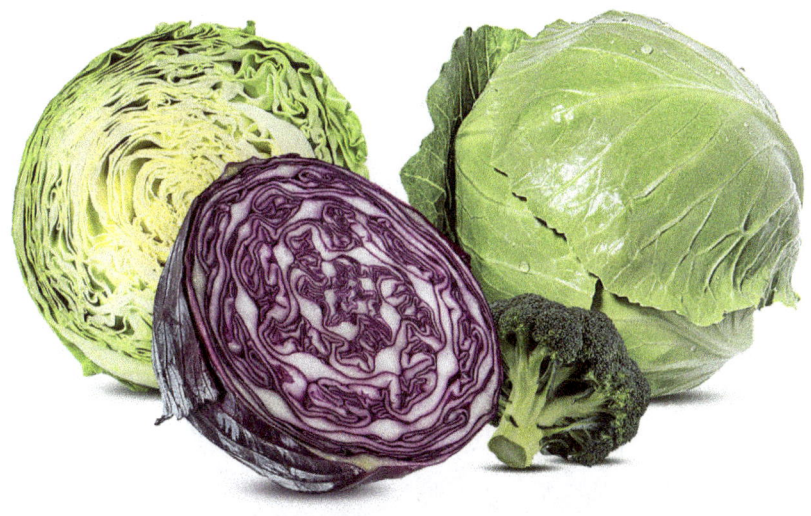

Cherries

A Sweet Way to Brighten Your Smile

Cherries are not just a delicious fruit—they can also aid in whitening your teeth naturally. Packed with antioxidants and vitamin C, cherries help reduce inflammation and support gum health. Their natural acidity can assist in breaking down surface stains on your teeth, while their high water content encourages saliva production, which helps cleanse your mouth and wash away food particles.

Incorporating cherries into your diet not only adds a sweet treat to your meals but also contributes to a brighter, healthier smile. Enjoy these vibrant fruits and let their natural properties enhance your oral care routine!

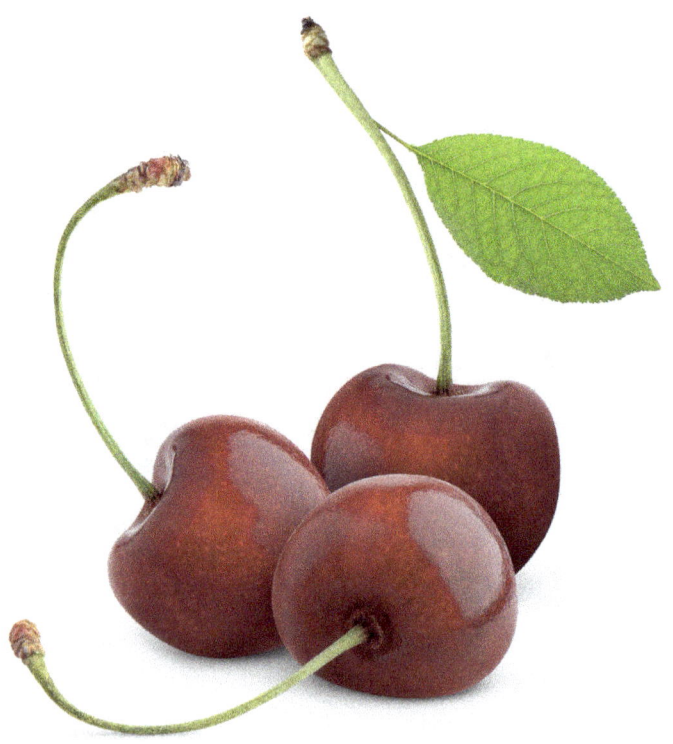

Cranberries

A Tart Twist to a Brighter Smile

Cranberries are not just a tangy treat—they also help naturally whiten your teeth. Rich in antioxidants and vitamin C, cranberries support gum health and protect against plaque buildup. Their natural acids can assist in breaking down surface stains, while the tartness stimulates saliva production, which helps wash away food particles and bacteria. Incorporating cranberries into your diet can contribute to a cleaner, brighter smile. Enjoy these vibrant berries in smoothies, salads, or as a refreshing snack, and let their natural properties enhance your oral health and brighten your teeth!

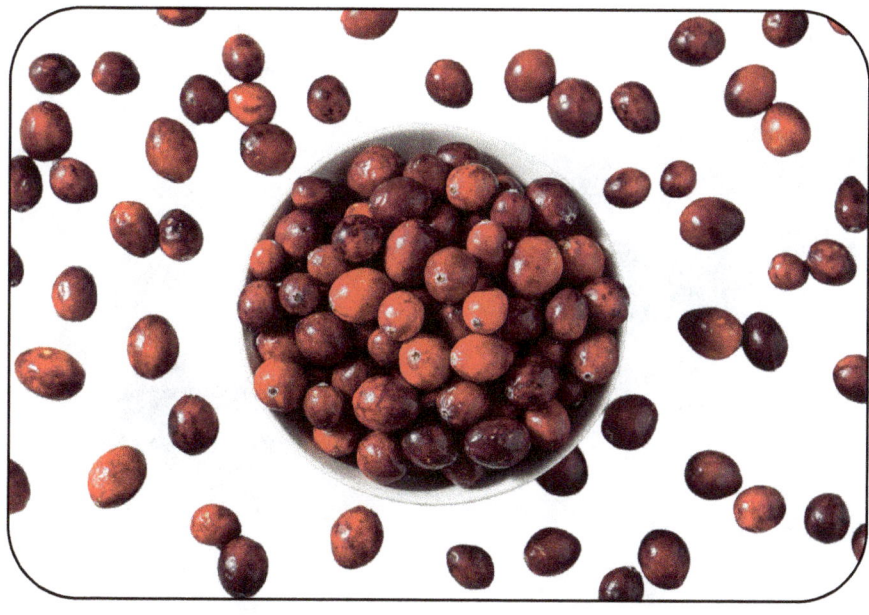

Cucumbers

A Refreshing Path to a Brighter Smile

Cucumbers are more than just a hydrating snack—they can also help whiten your teeth naturally. Their high water content aids in flushing out food particles and bacteria, promoting a cleaner mouth and reducing plaque buildup. The crisp texture of cucumbers stimulates saliva production, which further helps in naturally cleaning your teeth and preventing stains. Rich in vitamins and minerals, cucumbers also support overall oral health. Incorporating this refreshing vegetable into your diet can contribute to a brighter, healthier smile. Enjoy cucumbers in salads, sandwiches, or as a crunchy snack to reap the benefits for your teeth!

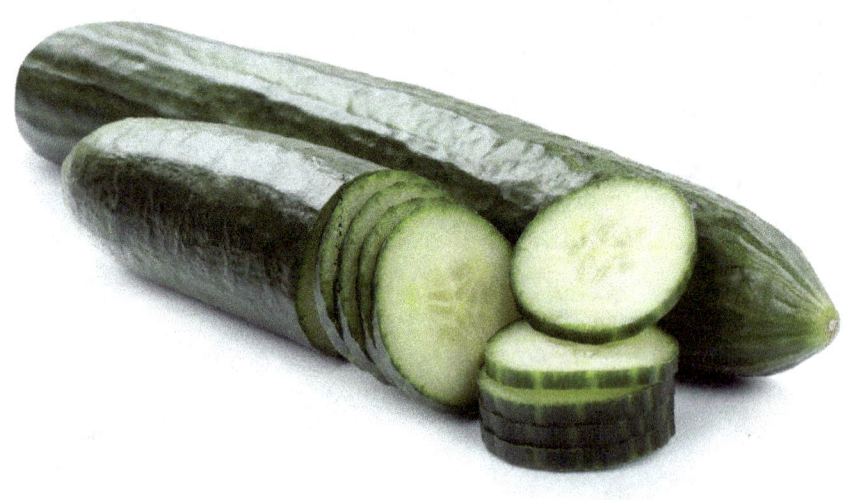

Candy

Sweet Tooth Truths

When you treat yourself to sweets, you're not just satisfying your sweet tooth—you're also exposing your teeth to potentially staining coloring agents. If you notice your tongue taking on an unusual color after indulging in candy, it's a sign that your teeth have probably been affected too.

Stay vigilant about the risk of tooth discoloration and choose moderation when enjoying sweets to maintain a vibrant and healthy smile.

Vogue nor WhiteBrights® has forecasted "purple tongues" becoming popular. Not this next season anyway. 😉

Side effects of smiling more will include increased happiness and contagious grins.

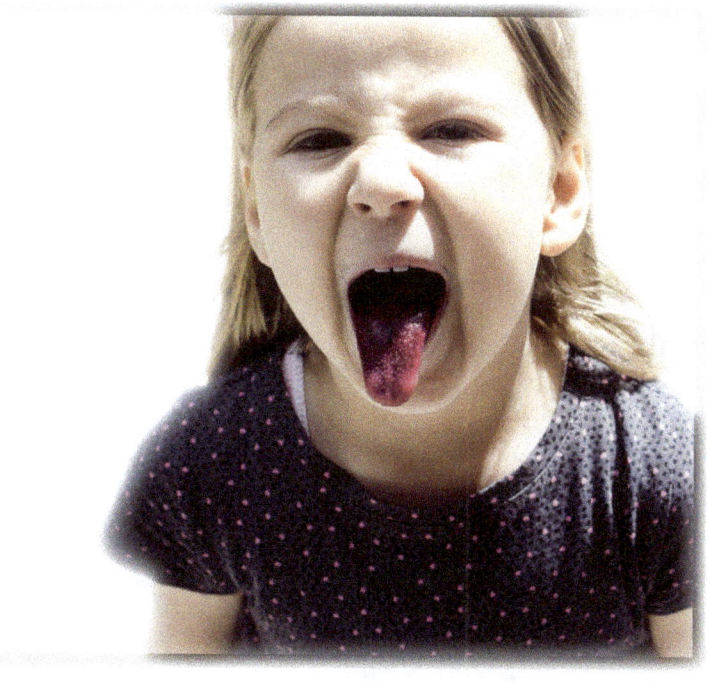

Cauliflower

Crunch Your Way to a Brighter Smile

With its crunchy texture, cauliflower works wonders as nature's way to crunch yourself to a brighter smile. It is effective at scrubbing away plaque buildup. Additionally, cauliflower stimulates saliva production, serving as a natural defense against stains adhering to your teeth.

Coarse vegetables like cauliflower and broccoli offer the most powerful whitening benefits when consumed raw. Their challenging texture requires thorough chewing, allowing the veggies to strip superficial stains from the tooth surface. Prolonged chewing promotes saliva production, aiding in the breakdown of stains for a brighter smile.

Carrots

The Carrot's role in Natural Whitening

Television's beloved talking horse, Mr. Ed, was onto something when he savored carrots. Packed with vitamin A, a crucial element in keratin—the protein responsible for fortifying tooth enamel — carrots play a vital role in maintaining dental health. Their crunchiness also offers tooth-whitening benefits.

Carrots, along with other crunchy vegetables like cucumbers, cauliflower, broccoli, and celery, serve as natural tooth whiteners. Their fibrous texture, when combined with saliva, effectively washes away food particles and stain-causing bacteria.

Beyond their eye-boosting properties, carrots serve as a versatile snack with numerous dental benefits. Each satisfying crunch helps remove plaque and stimulates saliva production, while also combating bad breath bacteria.

With their abrasive surface, raw carrots provide a quick and smooth polish for your teeth, making them an essential addition to your snack list.

Celery

Exploring the Smile-Boosting Powers of Celery

Celery, primarily composed of water, offers a refreshing treat that's beneficial to your smile. With each crisp bite, celery stimulates saliva production, promoting a neutralizing environment for bacteria and warding off cavities. In addition, its fibrous texture acts as a natural abrasive, effectively cleaning between teeth and providing a gentle massage for your gums. Incorporate celery into your snack routine for a refreshing and smile-enhancing treat.

Munch on crunchy celery and raw onions to naturally cleanse teeth and freshen breath. Their fibrous texture stimulates saliva production, which helps wash away stains and bacteria.

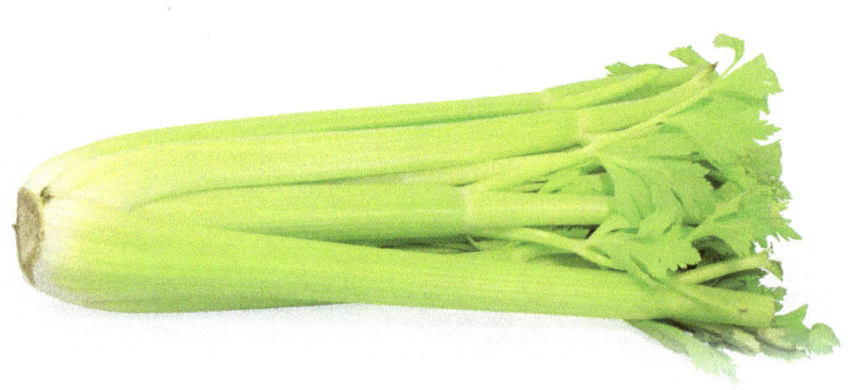

Crafting a Tooth-Friendly Charcuterie Board

Creating a charcuterie tray is the perfect time to have some fun with your food while keeping your teeth in top shape. Let's explore this charcuterie board that will wow your guests and keep your smile bright.

The Basics of Charcuterie

Charcuterie, pronounced "shahr-koo-tuh-ree," refers to the art of preparing and arranging cured meats, cheeses, fruits, and other accompaniments into a visually appealing and delicious spread. These appetizers are not only popular but with the right choices are also healthy and tooth-friendly.

Make It Healthy

Charcuterie boards can be as healthy or indulgent as you make them.

Here are some tips to ensure your board is kind to your smile

1. Start with Cheese

Cheese is the star of the charcuterie board and that is great news for your teeth! Rich in calcium, cheese helps remineralize tooth enamel and stimulate saliva production, which naturally cleans and protects your teeth. Opt for aged cheddar, Swiss, or Gouda, which have lower acidity levels. Arrange different shapes and varieties on a tray for a creative and interesting display.

2- Add Your Meats

Meat provides essential nutrients like protein and phosphorus, which support tooth enamel strength. While cured meats like salami and prosciutto are tasty staples, balance them with leaner options such as turkey or chicken breast to reduce salt and fat intake. Chewing meat also boosts saliva production, enhancing oral health.

3- Veggies

Incorporate vegetables like carrots, celery, and bell peppers. Their crisp texture acts as natural toothbrushes, scrubbing away food debris and plaque. Chewing these veggies stimulates your gums, improving blood circulation and overall gum health. They add vibrant color to your board and can replace starchy crackers and crisps.

4- Fruit

Add a touch of sweetness with fruits like apples, pears, and berries. While fruits contain natural sugars, their fibrous texture helps clean teeth and dislodge food particles. They also provide vitamins and antioxidants that support oral health. Highwater content fruits like apples and pears are especially beneficial.

5- Healthy Dips

Choose tooth-friendly dips to complement your board. Hummus, rich in calcium, and yogurt-based dips with probiotics are excellent choices. These dips promote strong teeth and a balanced oral microbiome, contributing to overall dental health.

6. Whole Grains

If including crackers or bread, opt for whole-grain varieties. Whole grains are packed with more nutrients and are less likely to stick to your teeth compared to refined grains. This reduces the risk of food particles lingering in your mouth.

7. Nutrient-Rich Nuts

Sprinkle nuts like almonds or walnuts into any gaps on your board. Nuts are crunchy, satisfying, and a great source of calcium and phosphorus, which help remineralize tooth enamel. They also add texture and visual appeal.

8. Unhealthy Additions to Avoid

To keep your charcuterie board tooth-friendly, steer clear of:

- Candies and Sugary Snacks: High sugar content feeds harmful bacteria, leading to tooth decay.
- Sticky or Hard Candies: Sticky candies promote plaque formation, and hard candies can chip or crack teeth.

9. Build Your Board

Crafting a tooth-friendly charcuterie board involves making thoughtful choices that delight your palate while protecting your dental health.

Cheese

Say Cheese! The Unexpected Culprit

When we think of a bright, white smile, cheese might not be the first food that comes to mind as a teeth whitening agent. However, it's a bit of a double-edged sword.

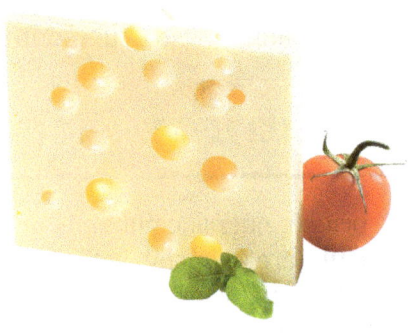

On one hand, cheese is rich in calcium and phosphorus, which can help strengthen tooth enamel and contribute to a whiter, brighter, healthier smile.

On the other hand, some cheeses, especially those with a more intense color, like cheddar, can contribute to staining.

The key lies in the amount and type of cheese you consume. The Smile Diet suggests opting for harder, paler cheeses as a safer bet for those looking to maintain a white smile. It's also recommended to enjoy cheese in moderation and to practice good oral hygiene by brushing or rinsing after indulging. By being selective with your cheese choices, you can enjoy this dairy delight without compromising your bright smile.

Hard cheeses, in particular, excel in dental care. Their firm texture aids in removing food particles, while their calcium content contributes to enamel strength. Incorporating dairy into your diet not only promotes oral health but also offers a natural defense against dental decay.

Unveiling the Cheesy Secrets for a Gouda Smile!

Hard cheese, those delightful little blocks often found on appetizer trays, are rich in calcium—a key ingredient for strengthening teeth and gums. Additionally, casein, a milk protein abundant in cheese, has been found to reduce the mineral loss you can experience from tooth enamel. Lactic acids present in cheeses play a vital role in protecting teeth against decay. Opt for a slice of aged gouda, known for its tough surfaces that can effectively remove stains caused by food particle buildup.

Recent studies suggest that incorporating cheese into your post-meal routine may help prevent tooth decay and promote enamel remineralization. Cheese contains proteins that inhibit harmful acids from binding to teeth.

A study in the journal General Dentistry found that cheddar consumption increased saliva production and formed a protective barrier on tooth enamel, resulting in pH level changes indicative of healthier teeth.

High in phosphate and calcium, cheese helps balance acidity levels in the mouth, warding off bacteria and preventing cavities and gum disease.

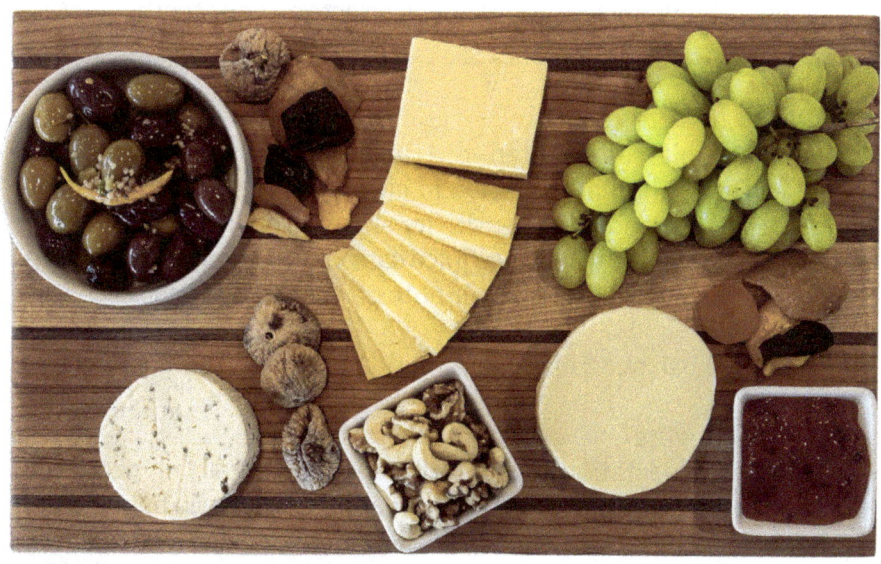

Citrus Squeeze

Freshening Your Smile

Turn up the brightness with citrus sensations! Lemons, oranges, and other citrus fruits contain natural acids that help whiten teeth, offering a zesty boost to your smile. These fruits are rich in vitamin C, which not only supports overall health but also stimulates saliva production. This increase in saliva helps wash away stains and bacteria, promoting a whiter smile and fresher breath.

> ## Nibble Knowledge - When you are craving something sweet
>
> We all crave a sweet treat from time to time. Enjoy your treat with a meal. Consuming sweets with meals prompts increased saliva production, which aids in neutralizing acid and washing away the food particles. This minimizes their staining effects on your teeth.

The Power of Citrus
While citrus fruits can brighten your smile, it's important to enjoy them in moderation. The natural acids in citrus can weaken enamel over time, potentially leading to sensitivity and erosion. A slice of lemon in your water or a splash of orange juice can be refreshing and beneficial, but overindulgence can put a sour note on your dental health.

Remember, a balanced diet is the foundation of a radiant smile!

Alkalizing Benefits
Contrary to expectations, citrus fruits possess alkalizing properties despite their high acid content. This means they can help balance your body's pH levels. Rich in vitamin C and bioflavonoids like hesperidin, citrus fruits contribute to bone health and overall well-being. These nutrients work together to support strong bones and teeth, highlighting the importance of whole foods in obtaining essential nutrients.

Key Points to Remember
- **Saliva Production:** Citrus fruits increase saliva production, which helps clean your mouth and maintain fresh breath.
- **Teeth Whitening:** The natural acids in citrus can aid in teeth whitening, but moderation is essential to avoid enamel erosion.
- **Bone Health:** Citrus fruits contain nutrients that support bone health, emphasizing the benefits of a balanced diet.

Enjoy the zest and benefits of citrus fruits, but always keep your dental health in mind. A little citrus can go a long way in maintaining a bright, healthy smile!

Citrus or Water?
Sip on water infused with a twist of lemon for a refreshing drink that can help naturally whiten teeth. The citric acid in lemons help remove surface stains over time.

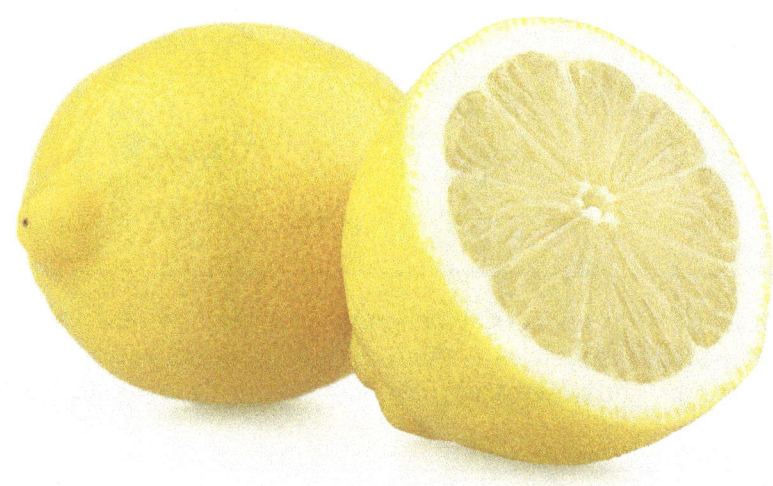

Citrus Lemon

A Citrus Wonder

When Life Gives You Lemons: Brighten Your Smile Naturally!

Does lemon whiten your teeth? "Just a Twist"

Lemons contain high acid level in the peel, which is a great whitener or even bleaching agent. You can use the lemon in two different ways; use the lemon peel to rub on your teeth or squirt the lemon juice on your teeth. If you decide to use the juice of the lemon you will need to mix it with an equal quantity of water.

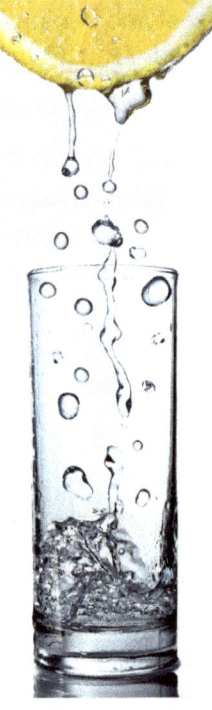

Fruits such as apricots, blueberries, oranges, peaches, pineapples, plums, and raspberries contain over 80% water. Melons such as cantaloupe and watermelon have some of the highest water content, at more than 90%.

Cinnamon

A Spicy Secret for a Whiter, Brighter Smile

In the quest for a dazzling smile, you might be surprised to learn that cinnamon, the spice often relegated to cozy lattes and holiday treats, can play a pivotal role in oral health and the pursuit of pearly whites. This aromatic spice is more than just a flavor booster—it's a potent ally for maintaining a healthy, radiant smile.

Whitening Wonders

Cinnamon contains natural compounds that can contribute to a whiter smile. Its mild abrasive texture helps remove surface stains from teeth, while its natural antibacterial properties help combat plaque buildup. Regular consumption or use of cinnamon-infused products can aid in maintaining a brighter smile by reducing the accumulation of discoloring agents on the enamel.

Oral Health Benefits

Beyond its whitening capabilities, cinnamon offers several benefits that promote overall oral health:

1. **Antibacterial Properties:** Cinnamon contains cinnamaldehyde, a compound with strong antibacterial effects that help reduce harmful bacteria in the mouth. This not only helps prevent cavities but also combats bad breath, leaving your mouth feeling fresh and clean.
2. **Anti-Inflammatory Effects:** The anti-inflammatory properties of cinnamon can help soothe gum inflammation and reduce the risk of gum disease. Regular use can help keep your gums healthy and your smile shining.
3. **Antioxidant Power:** Rich in antioxidants, cinnamon helps protect your teeth and gums from oxidative stress and damage. This can contribute to overall oral health and longevity, ensuring that your smile stays bright and youthful.

How to Incorporate Cinnamon into Your Smile Diet

Incorporating cinnamon into your daily routine can be as simple as adding a sprinkle to your morning oatmeal or smoothie. You can also enjoy cinnamon tea or chew on a cinnamon stick as a natural breath freshener. For those who prefer a more direct approach, consider using toothpaste or mouthwash containing cinnamon extract.

Conclusion

Cinnamon is a delicious and effective way to support oral health while working towards a whiter, brighter smile. By integrating this spice into your daily routine, you're not only enhancing your oral hygiene but also embracing a natural, holistic approach to maintaining your dental health. So next time you reach for your toothbrush, think of the spicy twist cinnamon can add to your smile care regimen and let its benefits spice up your path to a radiant grin.

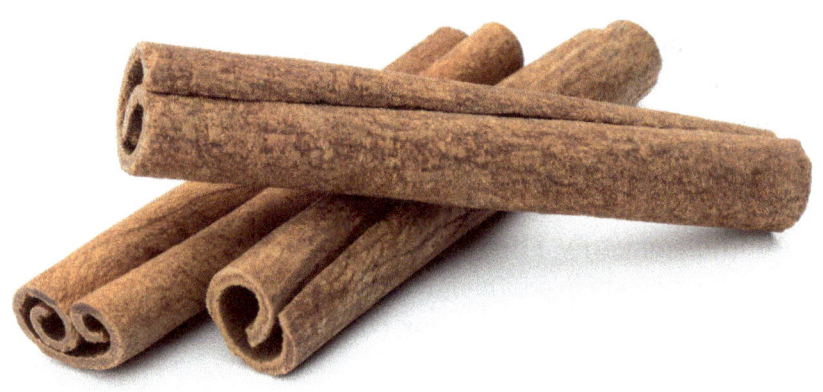

Clove

Nature's Secret for a Bright Smile

Clove is a superstar in the realm of dental care, famed for its powerful antiseptic properties, courtesy of eugenol, a key compound in clove oil. Research published in the Journal of Dentistry highlights clove oil's effectiveness against the bacteria responsible for dental plaque and bad breath.

How to Use Clove's for Oral Health
Step 1: Crush cloves into a fine powder.
Step 2: Mix the clove powder with a bit of olive oil to form a paste.
Step 3: Use this paste to brush your teeth, or simply chew on a clove for a few minutes.

Incorporating clove into your oral hygiene routine can help maintain a clean mouth, fresher breath and may contribute to whiter teeth over time.

Typically abrasive, lightly colored foods, like celery and carrots or even crunchy nuts and sesame seeds—nothing with dark pigments will help remove plaque naturally and can lighten the appearance of your teeth.

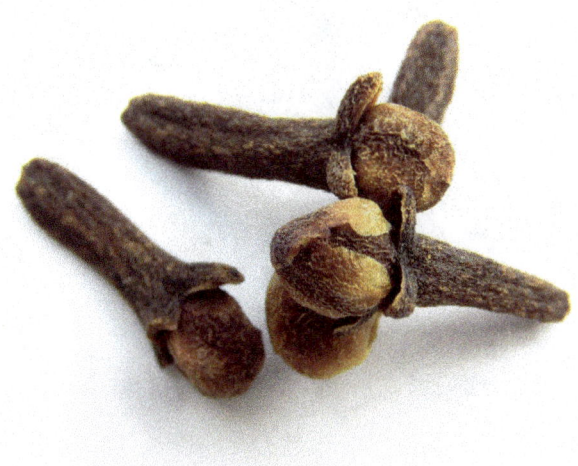

Cocoa

A Defender Against Dental Issues

Chocoholic's Delight: Discovering the Sweet Surprises of Cocoa for Your Smile!

Cocoa emerges as a potent combatant against gum inflammation and tooth erosion, both culprits in diminishing tooth whiteness. For best results, opt for darker chocolate, which typically contains less sugar, and is preferable for dental health.

The presence of cocoa in food appears to have a positive—or at least less detrimental—impact on tooth coloration. Incorporating cocoa into your diet may help defend against dental concerns, promoting a brighter and healthier smile. Compounds like theobromine found in dark chocolate may help harden enamel and reduce staining. Indulge in dark chocolate in moderation for potential tooth-stain prevention.

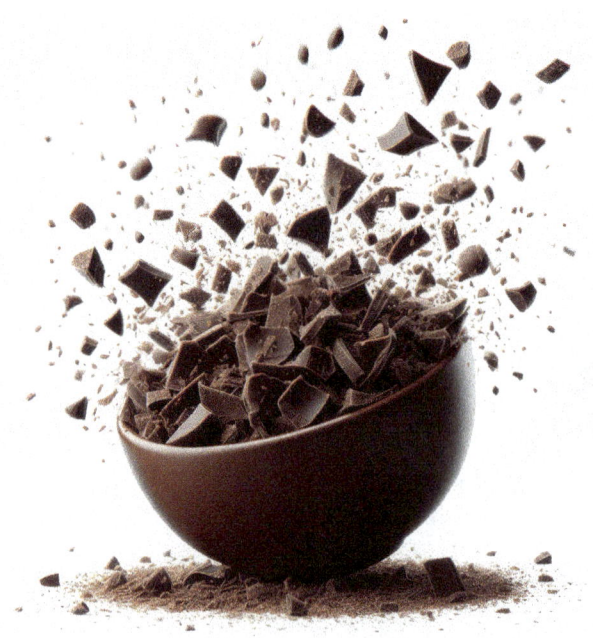

Coffee and Tea

Staining Culprits Brewing Duller Smiles

Americans Consume an Astonishing 146 Billion Cups of Coffee Annually

Similar to red wine, both coffee and tea contain tannins and phenolic acids that not only stain but can also damage your teeth. If you're a green tea enthusiast, opting for high-quality products may help mitigate discoloration to some extent.

Black Coffee and Tea: Darker Means More Staining

The deeper the hue of your beverage, the more prone it is to staining. Consider lightening the color by adding a splash of milk, which can help reduce the staining effect while still allowing you to enjoy your favorite brew.

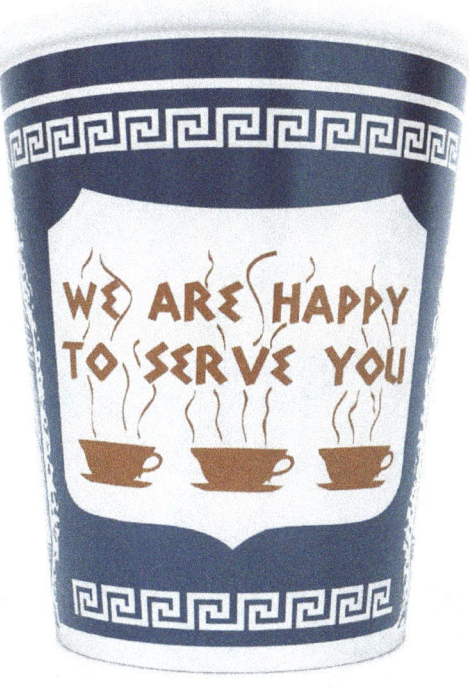

> By being aware of these staining foods and managing your diet, you can help preserve your teeth's natural whiteness.

> Small, inexpensive lifestyle changes can have a significant impact on your smile and oral hygiene.

> Fruits with a high water content clean plaque from your teeth and freshen your breath.

D

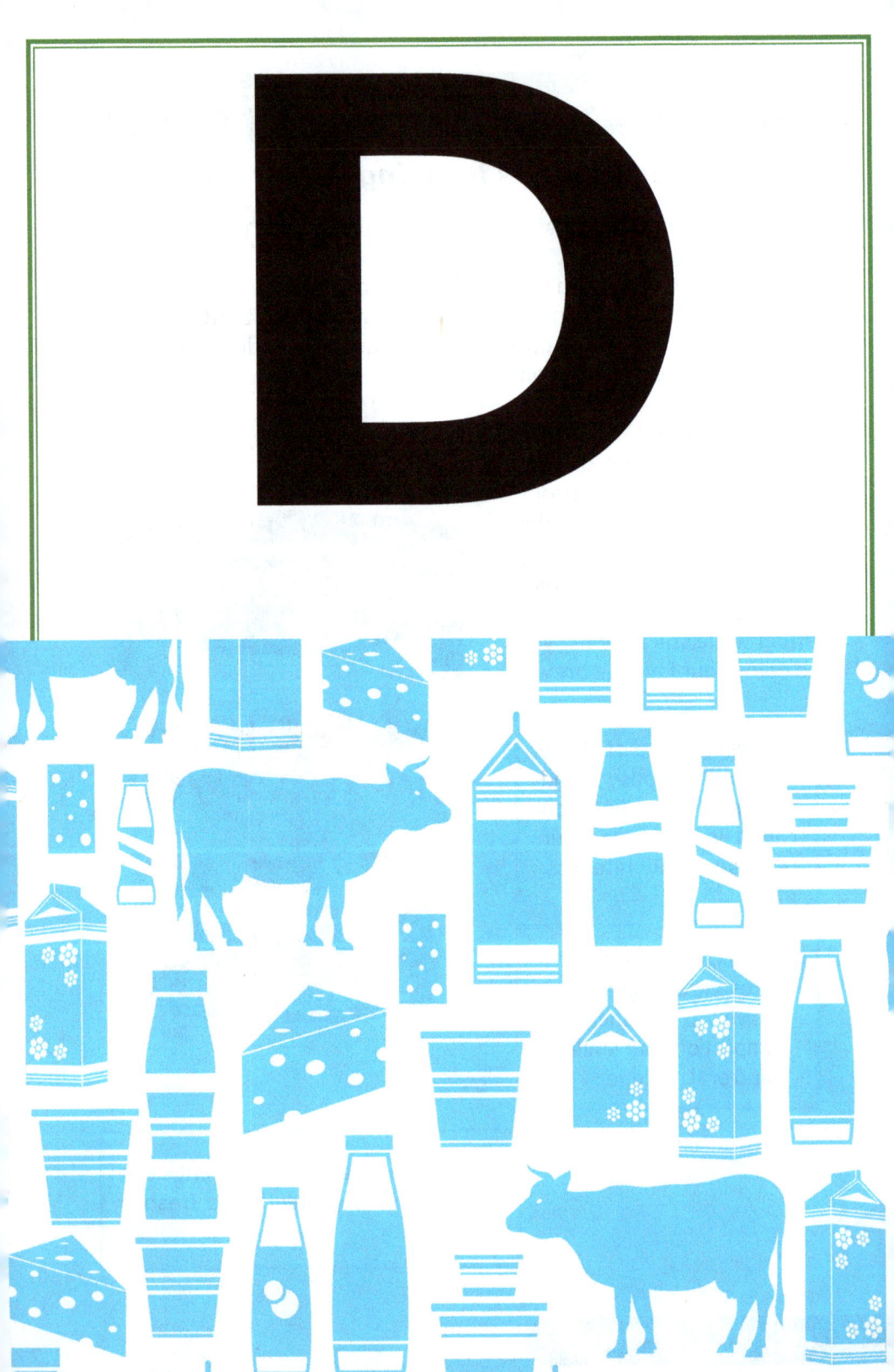

The Dairy Defense

Guardians of Dental Health

Uncover the teeth-whitening power of dairy delights! Incorporating dairy products into your diet not only boosts enamel strength but also contributes to overall dental health. Here's why:

- **Yogurt:** Rich in lactic acid and proteins, yogurt can create a protective barrier on your teeth, defending against harmful acids and bacteria.
- **Cheese:** Low-acidic cheeses like cheddar neutralize mouth acids and promote saliva production, which naturally cleans teeth and prevents cavities.
- **Calcium and Phosphorus:** These essential minerals found in dairy products are crucial for maintaining strong, healthy teeth and preventing discoloration.

Key Points to Remember

- **Protective Barrier:** Yogurt proteins may form a protective barrier on teeth, reducing the risk of cavities.
- **Acid Neutralization:** Cheeses help neutralize acids in the mouth, promoting a healthier oral environment.
- **Essential Minerals:** Calcium and phosphorus in dairy products strengthen enamel and protect against tooth decay.

Embrace the benefits of dairy for a brighter, healthier smile. Whether it's a serving of yogurt or a slice of cheese, your teeth will thank you for these delightful, nutritious additions to your diet.

If cow's milk cheese is a dental powerhouse, then goat cheese is a touchdown.

Avoid sweet potatoes and au gratin dishes, as they can stain your teeth. While rice and beans are popular, steer clear of black beans or any highly pigmented varieties to keep your smile bright.

E

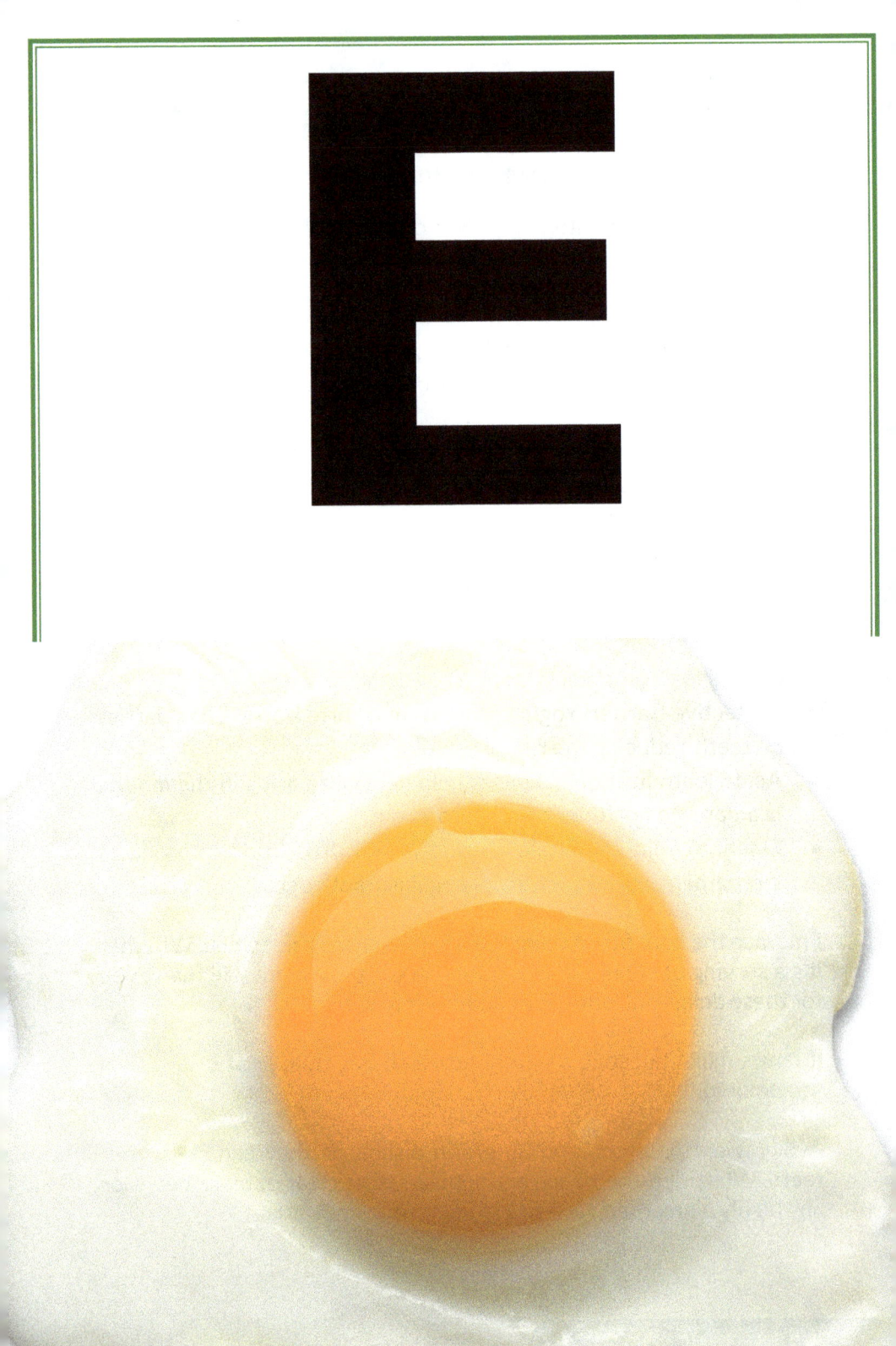

Edamame

A Bright Addition to Your Smile Diet

Edamame, those delightful young soybeans often served as a tasty appetizer, pack a powerful punch when it comes to supporting oral health and promoting a whiter smile. Here's why these little green gems are a fantastic addition to your Smile Diet:

Nutritional Powerhouse for Oral Health

1. **Rich in Calcium:** Edamame is a good source of calcium, which is crucial for maintaining strong teeth and bones. Calcium helps fortify tooth enamel, protecting against erosion and decay, and contributing to a healthier, brighter smile.
2. **High in Protein:** These soybeans are packed with high-quality protein, essential for the repair and regeneration of tissues in the mouth, including the gums. Healthy gums are foundational for a beautiful smile.
3. **Magnesium Content:** Edamame contains magnesium, a mineral that supports the absorption and metabolism of calcium, ensuring your teeth remain strong and resilient.
4. **Antioxidant Properties:** Edamame is rich in antioxidants like vitamin C and phytochemicals, which help combat inflammation and protect gum health. Healthy gums are vital for a radiant smile and the overall health of your mouth.
5. **Folate Benefits:** Edamame is a source of folate, a B vitamin that helps maintain the integrity of oral tissues and can reduce the risk of gum disease.
6. **Low Sugar Content:** Unlike many snacks that can contribute to tooth decay, edamame is low in sugar, making it a tooth-friendly option that won't harm enamel.

Edamame and Teeth Whitening
While edamame doesn't directly whiten teeth, its rich nutritional profile supports overall oral health, which is crucial for maintaining a white, bright smile. By strengthening enamel and promoting healthy gums, edamame helps create a mouth environment that is less conducive to staining and more supportive of whitening efforts.

Delicious and Versatile
Incorporating edamame into your diet is simple and delicious. Enjoy them steamed and lightly salted as a snack, toss them into salads, or blend them into hummus for a nutritious dip. Their versatility and mild flavor make edamame an easy way to boost your oral health.

Smile Tip: Pair edamame with foods high in vitamin D, like fish or fortified milk, to enhance calcium absorption and maximize benefits for your teeth.

Adding edamame to your diet not only contributes to overall health but also supports the maintenance of a vibrant, confident smile.

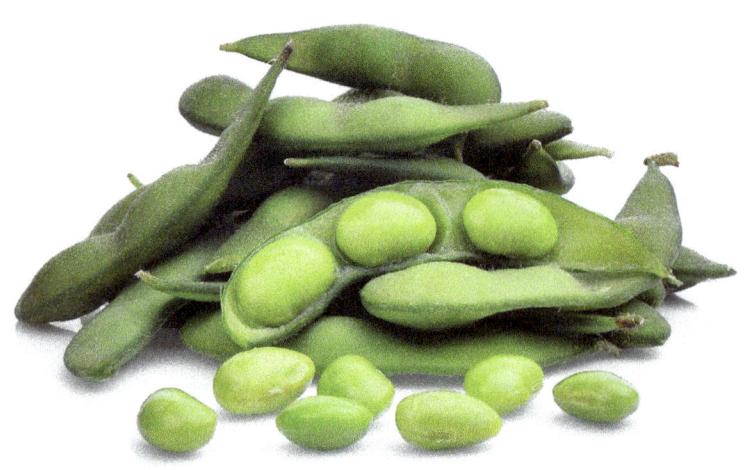

Echinacea

Nature's Boost for a Healthier Smile

Echinacea, a flowering plant known for its immune-boosting properties, offers surprising benefits for oral health and maintaining a bright smile. Here's how echinacea can be an ally in your journey to better teeth and gums:

Oral Health Benefits

1. **Anti-Inflammatory Properties:** Echinacea is renowned for its antiinflammatory effects, which can help reduce gum inflammation and support overall gum health. Healthy gums are essential for a bright, confident smile.
2. **Antimicrobial Effects:** The antimicrobial properties of echinacea may help combat harmful bacteria in the mouth, reducing the risk of plaque buildup and tooth decay. This can help keep your teeth clean and more resistant to discoloration.
3. **Immune Support:** By boosting the immune system, echinacea helps your body fight off infections, including those in the mouth. A strong immune system can help prevent gum disease and other oral health issues that can lead to tooth discoloration.
4. **Healing Support:** Echinacea can promote healing in oral tissues, making it beneficial for maintaining healthy gums and mucous membranes. Faster healing can help maintain a cleaner, healthier oral environment.
5. **Antioxidant Properties:** Rich in antioxidants, echinacea helps protect cells from damage and can support the health of tissues in the mouth. This protection is key to preventing oral health problems that could affect the appearance of your teeth.

Echinacea and Teeth Whitening

While echinacea doesn't whiten teeth directly, its ability to support gum health and reduce oral bacteria contributes to a cleaner, more vibrant smile. By keeping your mouth healthy, echinacea aids in maintaining the natural whiteness of your teeth.

How to Use Echinacea for Oral Health

- **Teas and Tinctures:** Echinacea teas and tinctures can be used as mouth rinses to take advantage of their antimicrobial properties. Simply swish the liquid in your mouth for a few minutes to help reduce bacteria.
- **Supplements:** Echinacea supplements can be taken to boost overall immune health, indirectly supporting oral health.
- **Toothpaste and Mouthwash:** Look for oral care products that contain echinacea extract as an ingredient to incorporate its benefits into your daily routine.

Smile Tip: Combine echinacea with other oral-friendly herbs like peppermint or chamomile to enhance its benefits and keep your mouth fresh.

Incorporating echinacea into your oral care routine can support healthier gums and teeth, contributing to a naturally brighter smile. Enjoy the holistic benefits of this powerful plant as part of your Smile Diet.

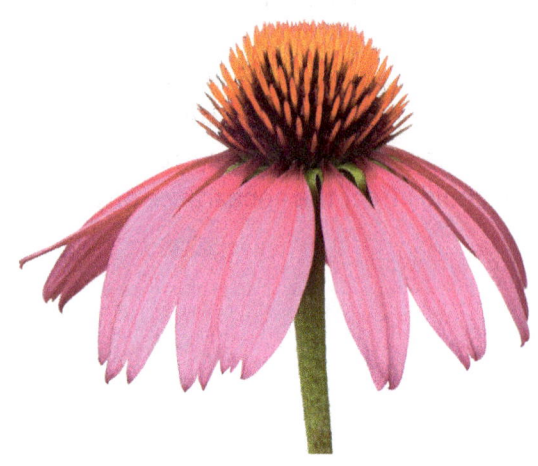

Eggs

Eggs can be a beneficial addition to your Smile Diet for teeth whitening and overall oral health for several reasons:

1. **Rich in Protein:** Eggs are an excellent source of high-quality protein, which is essential for maintaining the health of teeth and gums. Protein helps in the repair and regeneration of oral tissues.
2. **Calcium Content:** Eggs contain calcium, which is crucial for maintaining strong teeth and bones. Calcium helps protect the enamel, the hard outer layer of the teeth, from erosion and decay.
3. **Vitamin D:** Eggs are a good source of vitamin D, which is essential for calcium absorption in the body. Adequate vitamin D levels ensure that the calcium in your diet is effectively used to strengthen teeth and bones.
4. **Phosphorus:** Eggs also contain phosphorus, a mineral that works alongside calcium to strengthen teeth. Phosphorus is important for the formation of teeth and bones and helps repair the enamel.
5. **Antioxidants:** Eggs contain antioxidants like lutein and zeaxanthin, which may help reduce inflammation and support gum health. Healthy gums are essential for a bright smile and overall oral wellbeing.
6. **Protective Enzymes:** Some studies suggest that enzymes found in eggs, such as lysozyme, can help reduce harmful bacteria in the mouth, thereby reducing the risk of plaque buildup and tooth decay.
7. **Biotin:** Eggs are a source of biotin, a B vitamin that supports oral health by maintaining the mucous membranes in the mouth and aiding in the metabolism of fats, proteins, and carbohydrates.

When incorporating eggs into a diet aimed at teeth whitening and oral health, it's important to consider them as part of a balanced diet. They can be a valuable component of meals that promote strong, healthy teeth and contribute to a brighter smile.

Endive

The Crunchy Green for a Healthier Smile

Endive, a leafy green vegetable known for its crisp texture and slightly bitter taste, offers a range of benefits for oral health and teeth whitening. Incorporating Endive into your diet can support a healthier mouth and a brighter smile. Here's why this versatile vegetable is a great addition to your Smile Diet:

Nutritional Benefits for Oral Health

1. **Rich in Calcium:** Endive is an excellent source of calcium, which is essential for maintaining strong teeth and healthy enamel. A diet rich in calcium helps protect your teeth from erosion and decay, keeping them strong and bright.
2. **High in Fiber:** The high fiber content in endive stimulates saliva production, which is crucial for neutralizing acids and washing away food particles and bacteria. This natural cleansing action helps prevent tooth decay and discoloration.
3. **Vitamin K Content:** Endive contains vitamin K, a nutrient that plays a vital role in bone health and helps protect the integrity of oral tissues, including gums and enamel.
4. **Folate and B Vitamins:** Folate, along with other B vitamins found in endive, supports healthy gums by promoting cell growth and repair. Strong, healthy gums are essential for a radiant smile.
5. **Antioxidant Properties:** Endive is rich in antioxidants such as vitamin A and vitamin C, which help reduce inflammation and protect the gums from damage caused by free radicals. Healthy gums are less likely to recede, providing better support for teeth.
6. **Low in Sugar:** Endive is naturally low in sugar, making it a toothfriendly food that won't contribute to plaque buildup or cavities.

Endive and Teeth Whitening

While endive itself doesn't directly whiten teeth, its ability to support oral health creates a favorable environment for maintaining a bright smile. By promoting healthy gums and strong enamel, endive helps your teeth look their best naturally.

Delicious Ways to Enjoy Endive

- **Salads:** Add endive to salads for a crunchy, nutritious boost. Pair it with foods rich in vitamin C, like citrus fruits, to enhance its benefits.
- **Grilled or Roasted:** Enjoy endive grilled or roasted as a side dish to take advantage of its full flavor and nutritional benefits.
- **Dips and Wraps:** Use endive leaves as a low-calorie, tooth-friendly alternative to chips or bread for dips and wraps.

Smile Tip: Pair endive with foods high in vitamin D, such as eggs or mushrooms, to enhance calcium absorption and maximize benefits for your teeth and gums.

Incorporating endive into your diet not only contributes to your overall health but also supports the maintenance of a bright, confident smile. Enjoy the crisp, refreshing taste of endive while nourishing your teeth and gums.

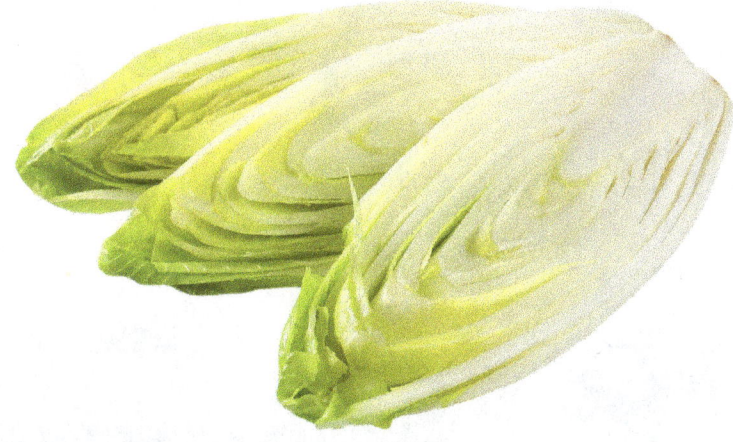

F

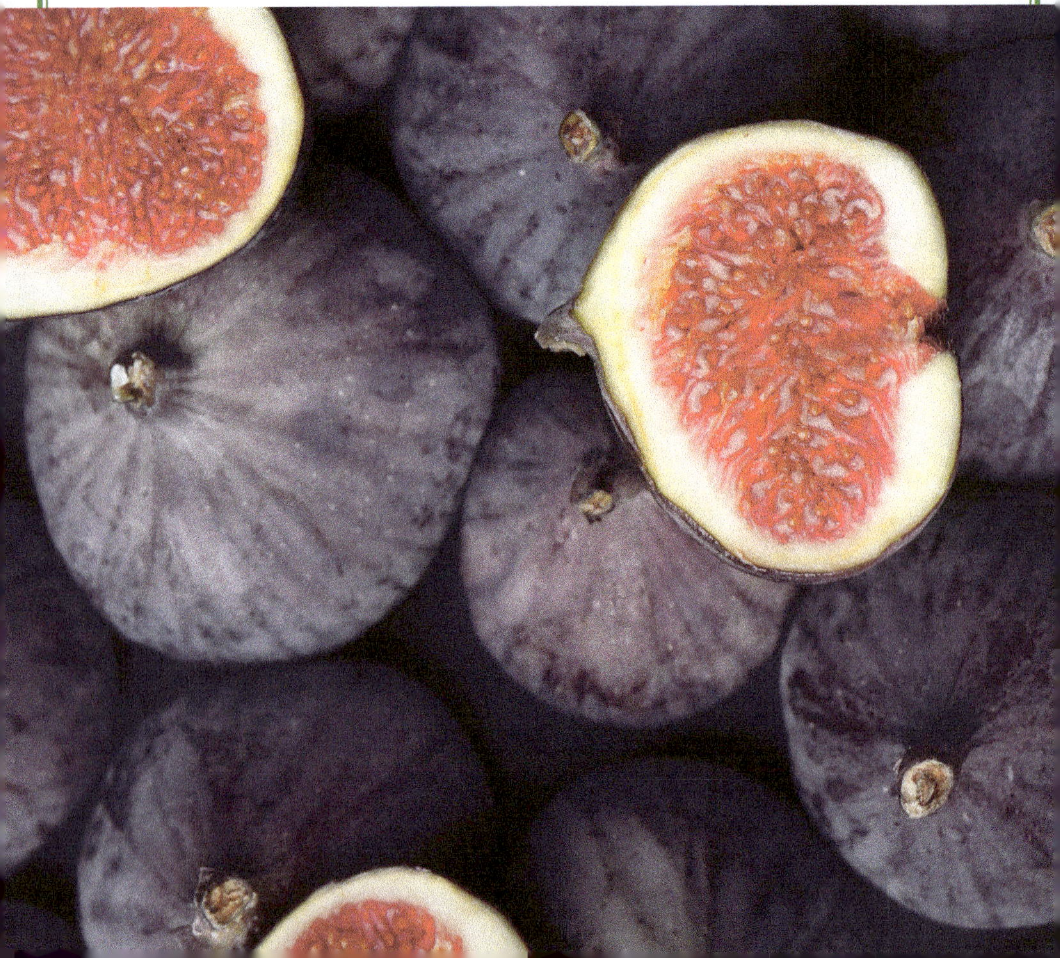

Figs

A Sweet Solution for a Brighter Smile

Figs are not just a delicious fruit—they can also help whiten your teeth naturally. Packed with dietary fiber, figs promote saliva production, which assists in cleansing your teeth and washing away food particles that can cause staining. Their natural sweetness and slight abrasiveness gently scrub away surface stains, contributing to a cleaner, brighter smile. Rich in essential vitamins and minerals, figs also support overall oral health. Enjoy these sweet, chewy fruits as a snack, or add them to your meals to enhance your oral care routine and brighten your smile naturally!

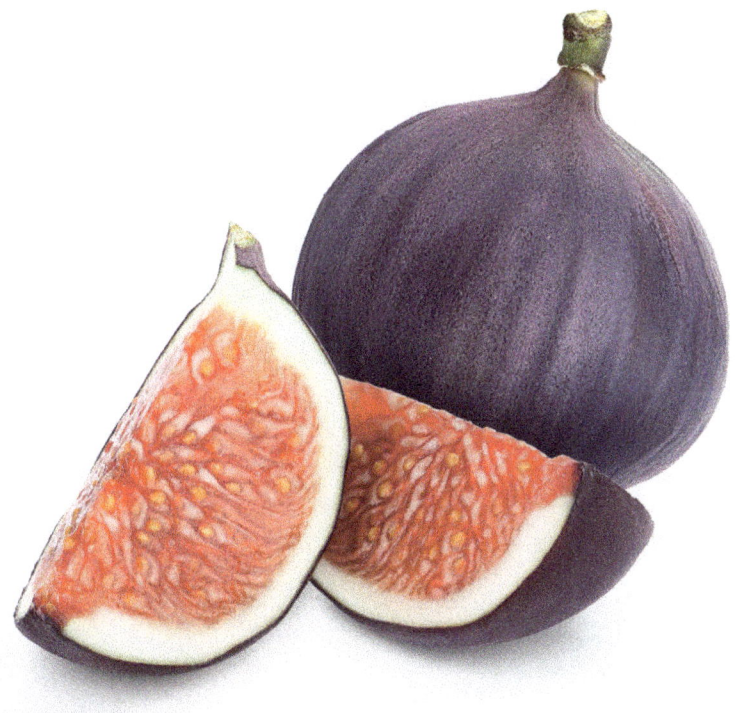

Fish

Reeling in the Benefits of Fish for Whiter Teeth!

Include seafood in your diet for another reason for a healthier mouth. Researchers at Harvard have found a connection between the omega-3 fatty acids present in fish and reduced rates of gum disease. Their hypothesis suggests that omega-3 fats might alleviate inflammation, such as redness and swelling, triggered by bacterial irritation in the gums.

Salmon is not only rich in calcium, which helps repair teeth but is also high in vitamin D which is essential for healthy bones and teeth.

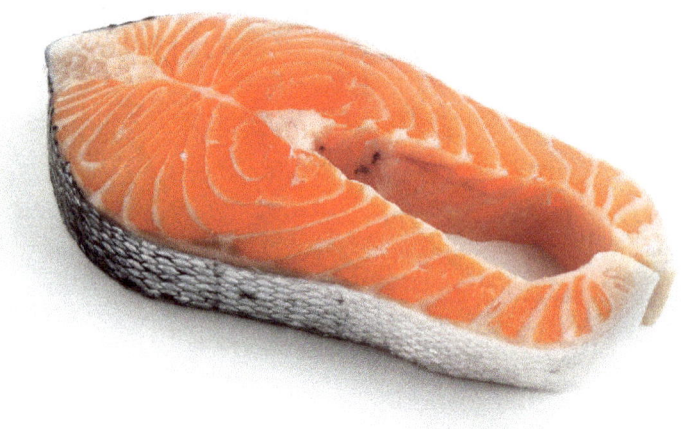

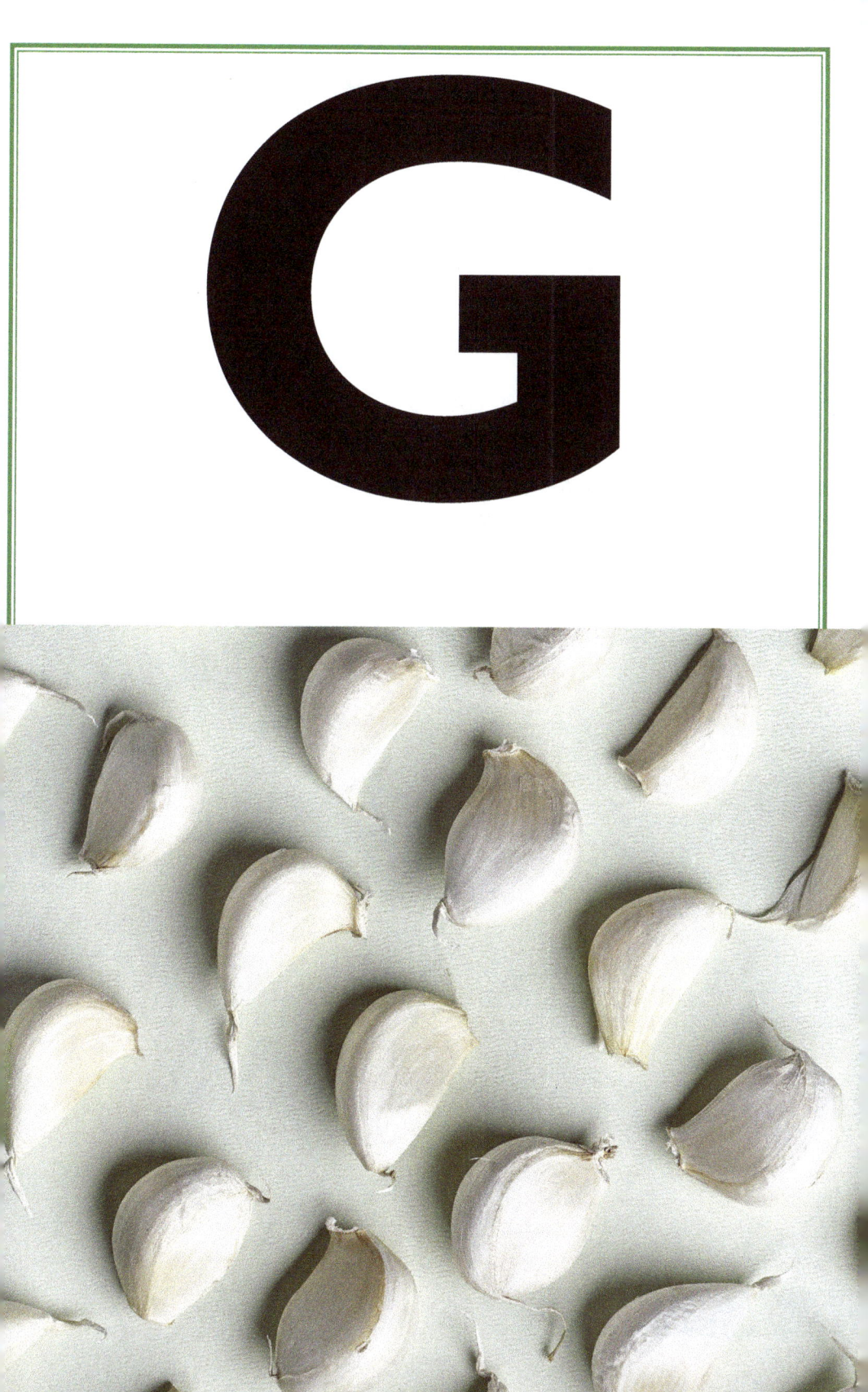

Garlic

The Power of Nature's Tooth Decay Fighter

Incorporating garlic into your diet can be a flavorful way to enhance your oral health and support teeth whitening efforts.

Whether added to meals or consumed raw, garlic offers a range of benefits that can contribute to a healthier, more radiant smile.

It is important to note that cooking garlic, like most everything else diminishes these beneficial properties.

For maximum benefits, incorporate raw garlic into your diet. Need I mention to "brush" for your loved one's comfort?

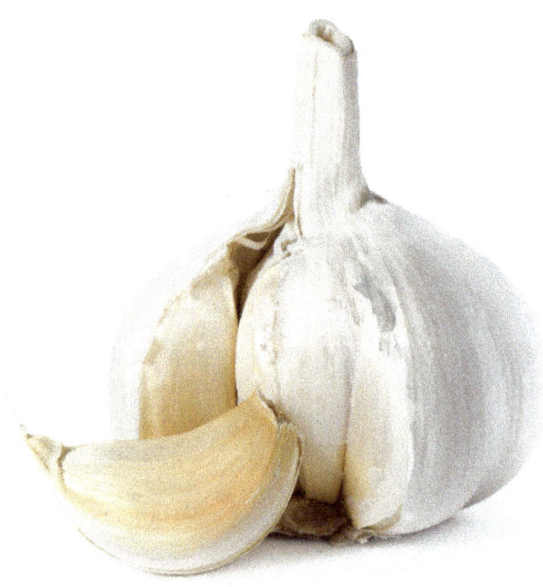

Ginger Root

Spice Up Your Smile:
Unveiling the Zesty Secrets of Ginger Root

The efficacy of ginger root in enhancing your oral health stems from its potent anti-inflammatory and antibacterial properties. Incorporating ginger into your diet can benefit individuals suffering from periodontitis, a condition characterized by inflammation leading to the deterioration of bone and connective tissue in the mouth.

By adding ginger to your meals, you not only introduce a delightful flavor but also harness its anti-inflammatory prowess, safeguarding against periodontal disease and promoting healthier gums and teeth.

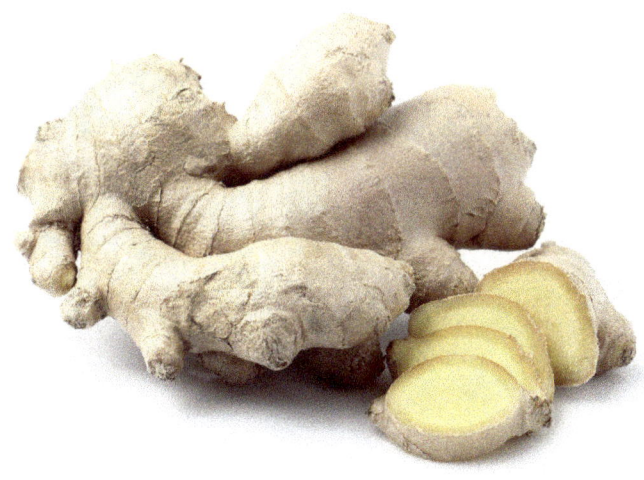

Grapes

A Juicy Boost for a Brighter Smile

Grapes are not only a tasty treat but also a natural aid for whitening your teeth. Their high water content helps wash away food particles and bacteria, reducing plaque buildup and preventing stains. Grapes contain antioxidants and natural acids that can help break down surface stains, while their crisp texture stimulates saliva production, which further cleanses your teeth. Including grapes in your diet supports a cleaner, brighter smile and enhances overall oral health. Enjoy these juicy fruits as a refreshing snack or add them to your meals for a naturally radiant smile!

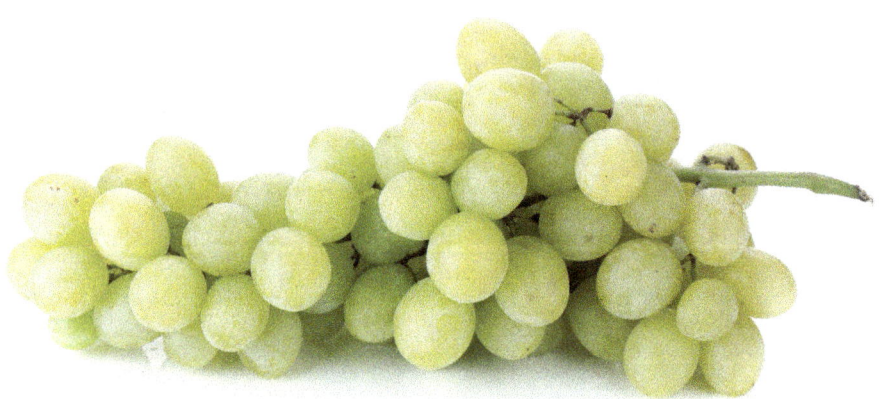

Green Tea

Sip and Smile: Unveiling the Brightening Powers of Green Tea!

With its lighter hue, green tea is less likely to stain your teeth, offering a promising solution for those seeking a radiant smile.

Beyond its cosmetic benefits, green tea also provides significant advantages for oral health.

A comprehensive study conducted in 2009 evaluated the periodontal well-being of 940 men, revealing a noteworthy correlation between regular green tea consumption and improved teeth and gum health.

The findings showed that individuals who incorporated green tea into their daily routine exhibited healthier teeth and gums compared to those who didn't.

Remarkably, for each additional cup of green tea consumed daily, there was a discernible reduction in markers associated with tooth and gum diseases. Embrace the refreshing taste of green tea not only for a brighter smile but also for your overall dental wellness.

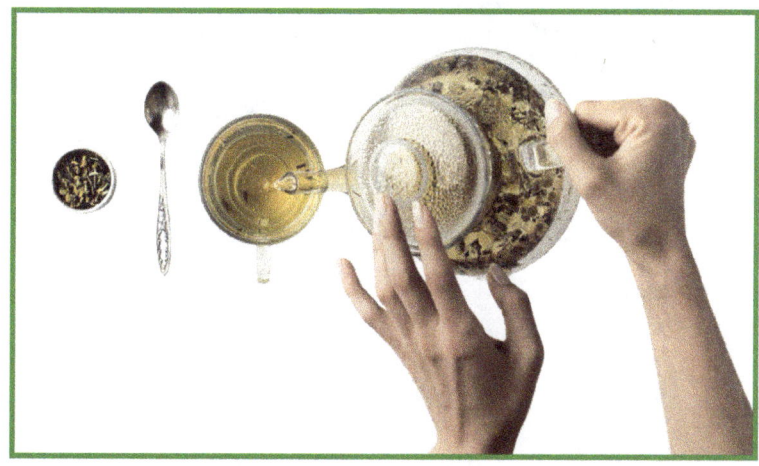

Green Beans

A Crisp Ally for a Brighter Smile

Green beans are more than just a nutritious vegetable—they also help naturally whiten your teeth. Their crunchy texture stimulates saliva production, which aids in cleansing your teeth and washing away food particles that can lead to stains. The high fiber content of green beans helps reduce plaque buildup and supports overall oral health. Rich in vitamins and minerals, green beans contribute to strong enamel and a brighter smile. Incorporate this crisp vegetable into your meals for a tasty way to enhance your oral care routine and promote a naturally whiter smile!

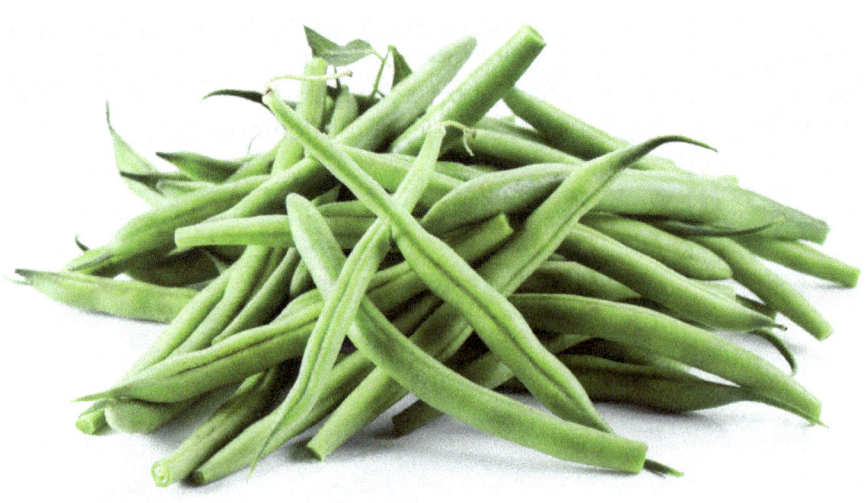

Guava

A Tropical Treat for a Brighter Smile

Guava is not just a delicious tropical fruit—it also aids in naturally whitening your teeth. Packed with vitamin C and antioxidants, guava supports gum health and helps reduce plaque buildup, which can contribute to stains. Its high fiber content stimulates saliva production, which assists in cleansing your teeth and removing surface stains. Additionally, the natural acidity of guava can gently break down discoloration. Enjoy this vibrant fruit as a refreshing snack or add it to your meals to boost your oral care routine and achieve a naturally whiter, healthier smile!

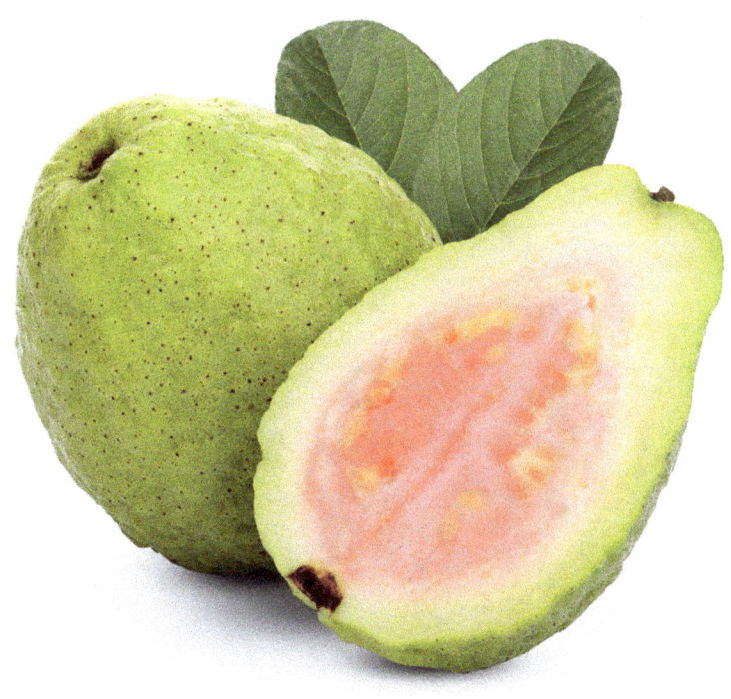

GUM

Chew on This: Gum's Secret Benefits for a Brighter Smile!

Chewing gum, specifically sugarfree varieties, can be a real boon for your dental health. After meals, chewing a piece of sugar-free gum stimulates saliva production, effectively rinsing away bacteria and neutralizing acid residues from your food intake.

Opt for gums containing xylitol, which is specifically known to combat bacteria and thwart plaque formation.

Sugar-free gum doesn't just freshen your breath; it can also aid in cleaning teeth, particularly in situations where brushing isn't immediately feasible.

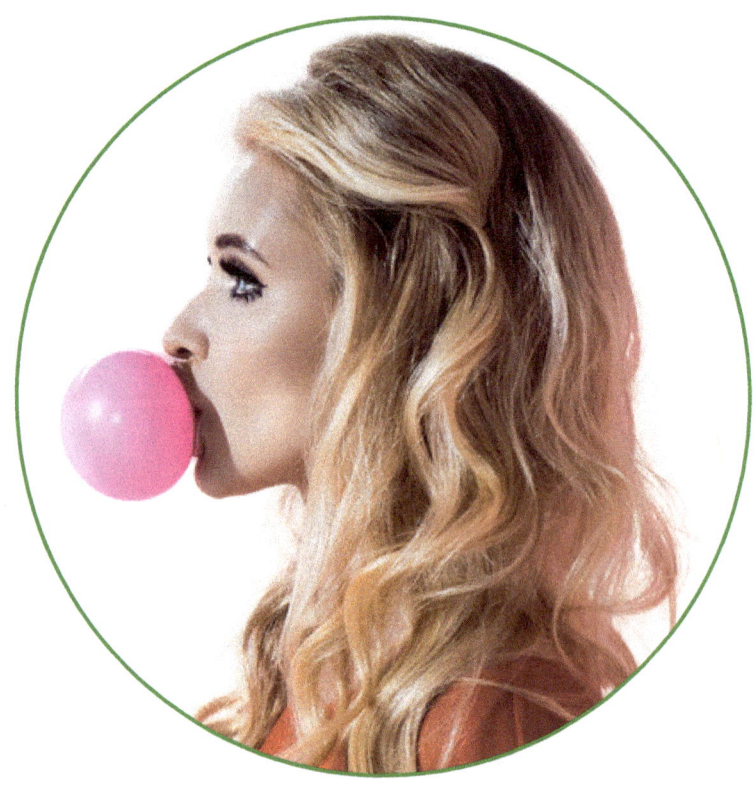

Nibble Knowledge

Smile Diet Tip- Satisfy Sweet Cravings with Sugarless Gum

When those sweet cravings strike, reach for sugarless gum as your go-to option! Just like having a trusty friend by your side, keeping sugarless gum readily available ensures you have a satisfying solution at hand whenever the urge for sweetness arises.

Chewing sugarless gum for 20 minutes after eating foods with high acid content will assist you in deterring the harmful effects of the food.

Who recalls the days of Bubble Yum and Hubba Bubba? Ah, the nostalgia! Even before Bubble Yum disappeared from the checkout aisles, they introduced a sugarless version. Research suggests that chewing sugarless gum can boost feelings of fullness, making it a handy tool to help lose weight.

After a meal, if brushing isn't an immediate option, chewing sugarless gum can also help by stimulating saliva production, aiding in removing food particles and acidic residues from your mouth.

So, next time you crave something sweet, pop in a piece of sugarless gum and keep that smile on your face as you stay on track with your smile diet!

Gummy Vitamins

A Sticky Situation for Your Smile

They're good for you, right? Maybe for your health, but not so much for your teeth. These chewy supplements can be a trifecta of trouble for your smile.

Here's why

First, gummy vitamins are packed with sugar, which can wear down your tooth enamel, making it more prone to discoloration.

When your enamel is worn down, your teeth become more susceptible to decay, leading to cavities and other dental issues.

Then there's the sugar. Bacteria in your mouth feed on sugar and produce even more acid. This acid further softens your enamel, increasing the risk of decay and cavities.

To make matters worse, gummy vitamins tend to stick to your teeth. This means the sugar and citric acid can linger in your mouth longer, giving them more time to cause damage.

While gummy vitamins might be a sweet and convenient way to get your nutrients, they're not so kind to your teeth.

To keep your smile bright and healthy, consider alternative vitamin options that are less harmful to your teeth.

If you decide to indulge, make sure to brush your teeth or rinse your mouth with water afterward.

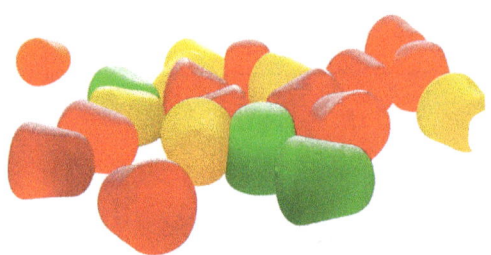

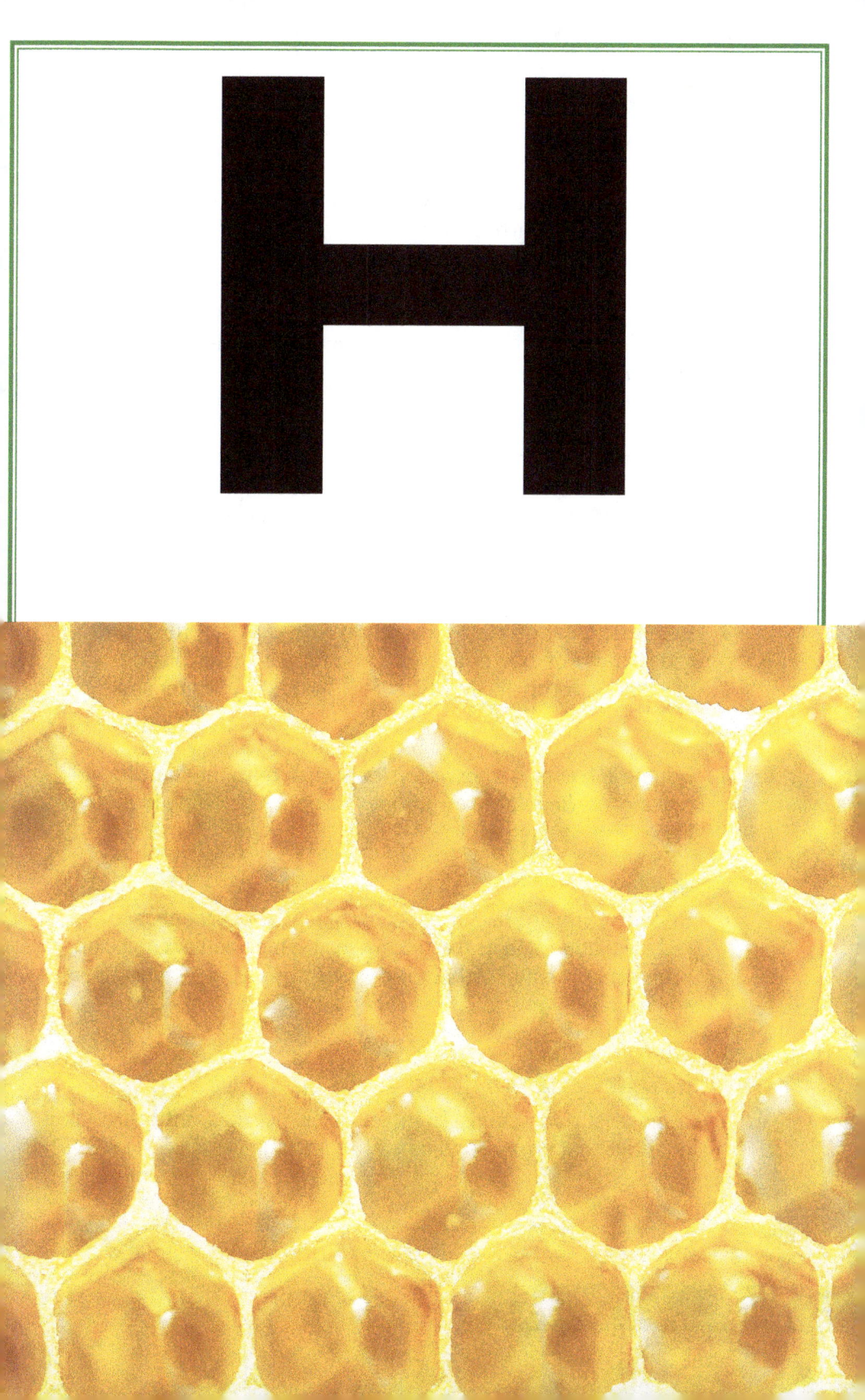

Herbs

Here's a list of herbs that are known for their benefits in teeth whitening and overall oral health:

1. **Basil**
   - **Benefits:** Basil leaves have natural teeth-whitening properties and can help in maintaining oral hygiene. It's also effective in preventing bad breath.

2. **Clove**
   - **Benefits:** Clove has strong antibacterial properties and can help in reducing bacteria in the mouth that cause tooth discoloration. It's also great for overall oral health, helping with toothache and gum issues.

3. **Licorice Root**
   - **Benefits:** Licorice root has compounds that can help inhibit the growth of bacteria in the mouth, reducing plaque and preventing tooth decay, which contributes to a whiter smile.

4. **Neem**
   - **Benefits:** Neem is known for its antibacterial and antifungal properties. Regular use can help prevent plaque buildup and keep teeth looking whiter.

5. **Peppermint**
   - **Benefits:** The antibacterial properties of peppermint can help reduce plaque, and its fresh scent makes it a popular choice for promoting fresh breath, indirectly contributing to a brighter smile.

6. **Sage**
   - **Benefits:** Sage has natural astringent properties that help remove surface stains from teeth. It also has antibacterial qualities that promote gum health.

7. **Thyme**
    - **Benefits:** Thyme has antiseptic and antibacterial qualities that help prevent tooth decay and gingivitis, keeping your smile healthy and bright.

8. **Turmeric**
    - **Benefits:** Despite its vibrant color, turmeric has been used traditionally for whitening teeth due to its anti- inflammatory and antibacterial properties, which help in reducing plaque and inflammation.

Incorporating these herbs into your diet or oral care routine can naturally support teeth whitening efforts and improve overall oral health.

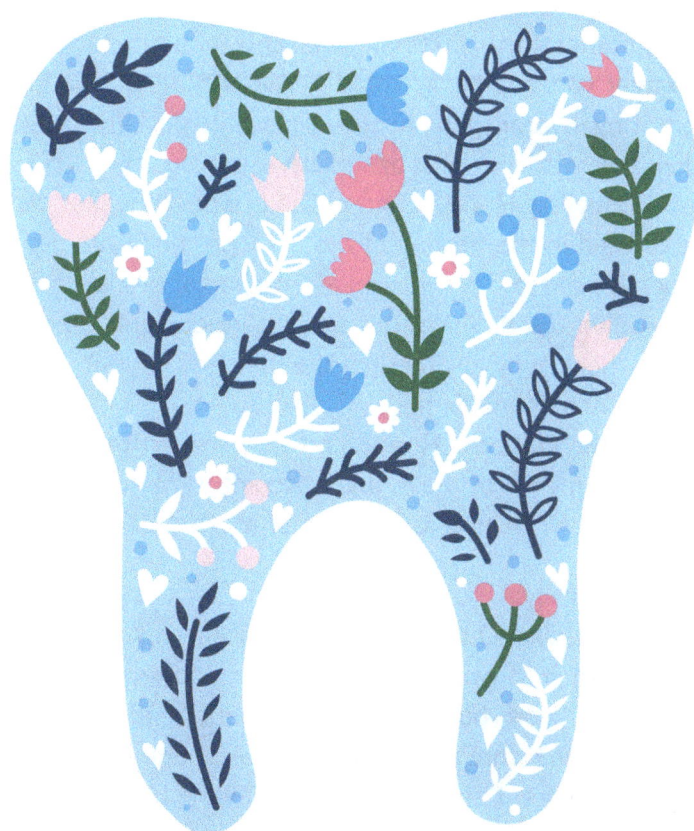

Honey

A Sweet Solution for Oral Health

Honey is not only a delicious natural sweetener but also offers some surprising benefits for oral health. While it's important to consume honey in moderation due to its sugar content, certain properties of honey can promote a healthy mouth. Here's how honey can contribute to your teeth and gums:

1. **Antibacterial Properties:** Honey has natural antibacterial properties, particularly when it comes to fighting oral bacteria that can lead to cavities and gum disease. This helps in reducing plaque buildup, which can otherwise lead to tooth discoloration and decay.
2. **Anti-inflammatory Effects:** The anti-inflammatory properties of honey can soothe irritated gums and reduce inflammation, promoting overall gum health. This is especially beneficial for individuals with gingivitis or sensitive gums.
3. **Wound Healing:** Honey is known for its wound-healing capabilities and can aid in the healing of mouth sores or ulcers. Its soothing properties can also provide relief from minor oral irritations.
4. **Antioxidant Content:** Honey contains antioxidants that contribute to oral health by protecting the tissues in your mouth from oxidative stress and damage.
5. **Natural Moisturizer:** Honey can help retain moisture in your mouth, reducing dryness and discomfort associated with dry mouth, which can increase the risk of tooth decay and bad breath.

Using Honey Safely:

- **Rinse After Use:** Due to its sugar content, it's essential to rinse your mouth with water after consuming honey to prevent sugar from lingering on your teeth and contributing to decay.
- **Choose Raw Honey:** Opt for raw or Manuka honey, which may offer more potent antibacterial and healing properties compared to processed varieties.

- **Moderation is Key:** Enjoy honey as part of a balanced diet and ensure proper oral hygiene practices, including regular brushing and flossing, to maintain your dental health.

While honey alone won't whiten your teeth, its antibacterial and antiinflammatory properties can support overall oral health, creating a cleaner environment that helps maintain your natural tooth color.

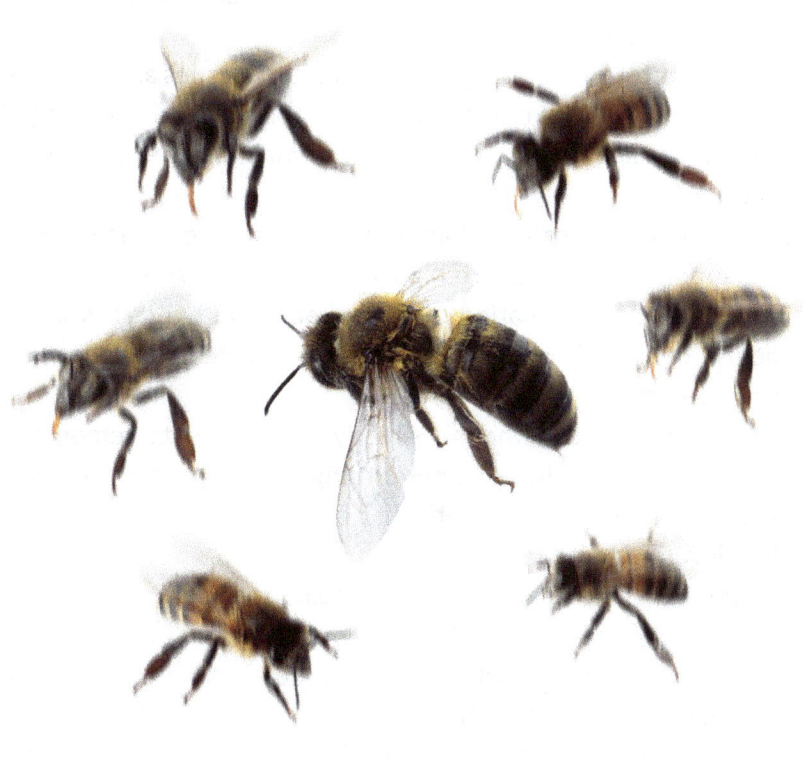

Hummus

A Savory Treat for Oral Health

Hummus, a creamy blend of chickpeas, tahini, olive oil, lemon juice, and garlic, is not just a delicious snack but also beneficial for your oral health. Here's how incorporating hummus into your diet can support teeth whitening and overall gum health:

1. **Rich in Phosphorus:** Chickpeas, the main ingredient in hummus, are rich in phosphorus, a mineral essential for maintaining healthy teeth and bones. Phosphorus works alongside calcium to keep your tooth enamel strong, which is crucial for protecting against decay and discoloration.
2. **High in Protein:** Protein is vital for repairing tissues and promoting healthy gums. A diet rich in protein supports overall oral health by helping to regenerate gum tissue and maintain the structure of your teeth.
3. **Antioxidant Properties:** Hummus contains ingredients like garlic and lemon juice, which are high in antioxidants. Antioxidants can help reduce inflammation and combat oxidative stress in your mouth, contributing to healthier gums and reducing the risk of oral diseases.
4. **Alkaline-Forming:** Although slightly acidic due to lemon juice, hummus is generally alkaline-forming once digested, helping to neutralize acids in the mouth that can erode enamel and lead to discoloration.
5. **Supports Saliva Production:** The combination of flavors in hummus can stimulate saliva production, which is crucial for washing away food particles and bacteria, reducing plaque buildup, and maintaining a naturally whiter smile.
6. **Low in Sugar:** Hummus is naturally low in sugar, which helps prevent the growth of cavity-causing bacteria and minimizes the risk of tooth decay.

Incorporating Hummus into Your Diet:
- **Healthy Snack:** Enjoy hummus as a healthy snack with crunchy vegetables like carrots or celery, which can further aid in cleaning your teeth naturally.
- **Balanced Diet:** Pair hummus with a balanced diet that includes other oral health-friendly foods to maximize the benefits for your teeth and gums.
- **Oral Hygiene:** While hummus can support oral health, it's important to maintain regular oral hygiene practices, including brushing twice a day and flossing, to keep your smile bright and healthy.

Hummus, with its nutrient-rich ingredients, is a tasty and healthful addition to your diet that supports strong teeth and healthy gums, contributing to a brighter and healthier smile.

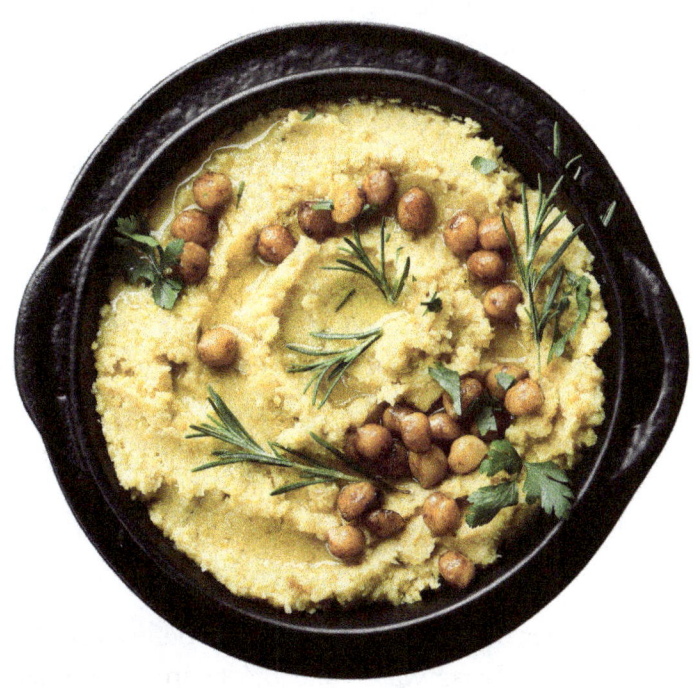

Hydrogen Peroxide

A Powerful Ally for Teeth Whitening

Hydrogen peroxide is widely recognized for its teeth-whitening properties and is a common ingredient in many dental products. However, Hydrogen peroxide should be used with caution and not swallowed.

Here's how hydrogen peroxide can contribute to whiter teeth and support oral health:

1. **Effective Whitening Agent:** Hydrogen peroxide is a natural bleaching agent that can help remove stains from the surface of your teeth. It works by breaking down the molecules that cause discoloration, resulting in a brighter, whiter smile.
2. **Antibacterial Properties:** Hydrogen peroxide is known for its ability to kill bacteria, making it effective in reducing the number of harmful bacteria in the mouth. This helps prevent plaque buildup and reduces the risk of gum disease.
3. **Prevents Bad Breath:** By killing odor-causing bacteria, hydrogen peroxide can help reduce bad breath, contributing to fresher breath and improved oral hygiene.
4. **Gum Health Support:** While hydrogen peroxide can be beneficial for gum health due to its antibacterial properties, it should be used with caution. Diluted solutions can help soothe minor gum irritations, but it's important to avoid prolonged use to prevent irritation.
5. **Reduces Gum Inflammation:** The antibacterial action of hydrogen peroxide can help reduce gum inflammation caused by bacterial infections. However, it should be used carefully to avoid irritation.

Using Hydrogen Peroxide Safely:

- **Dilution:** Always dilute hydrogen peroxide before use. A common mixture is equal parts water and 3% hydrogen peroxide. This reduces the risk of irritation to your gums and enamel.

- **Mouthwash:** Use the diluted solution as a mouthwash, swishing it around your mouth for about 30 seconds before spitting it out. Avoid swallowing.
- **Whitening Paste:** You can mix hydrogen peroxide with baking soda to create a paste for brushing. However, use this sparingly as it can be abrasive and potentially damage enamel if used too frequently.
- **Professional Guidance:** Consider consulting with a dentist before using hydrogen peroxide for teeth whitening, especially if you have sensitive teeth or existing dental issues.

⚠️ The Hydrogen Peroxide Warning: Proceed with Caution!

While hydrogen peroxide can be used for teeth whitening, **using it at home without professional supervision can be risky.** Overuse or improper concentration can lead to **enamel erosion, gum irritation, and increased tooth sensitivity.** Plus, DIY methods using straight Hydrogen Peroxide lack the precise formulation needed for **safe and effective whitening**—leaving you with unpredictable results (and possibly a frown instead of a brighter smile).

A Smarter, Safer Way to Whiten
Instead of taking unnecessary risks, opt for a professional at-home whitening kit or consult with your dentist for expert care. At WhiteBrights.com, where we take whitening seriously. Our SAFE-T PROMISE guarantees a whitening experience that is:

- ✅ **S**-SAFE
- ✅ **A**-AFFORDABLE
- ✅ **F**-FAST ACTING
- ✅ **E**-EFFECTIVE
- ✅ **T**-TEAR (PAIN) FREE

<u>www.WhiteBrights.com</u> for 25% off your first order—a little reward for reading my book and choosing a safer, more effective way to brighten the world with your smile.

Always *Stay Smilin!*

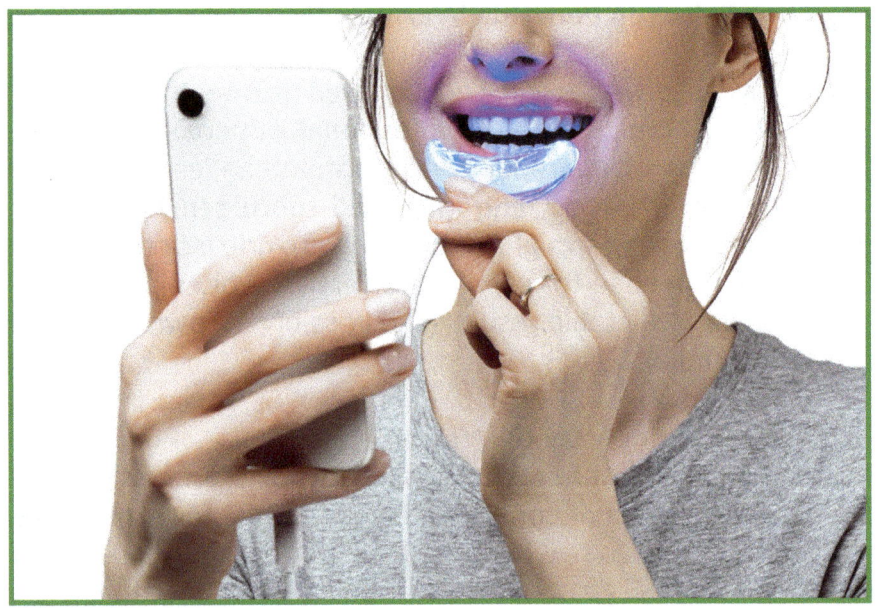

Hydrate for Health

Choose Fluorinated Water

In your journey towards a radiant smile and a healthier you, hydration is key. Opting for fluorinated water not only quenches your thirst but also acts as a shield against tooth decay.

Roughly 73% of the U.S. population with public water access in 2020 received drinking water with fluoride.

Whether you're sipping from the tap or grabbing a bottle, take a moment to check the label. Look for the fluoride content to ensure you're getting that extra boost in dental protection. With each sip, you're not just hydrating your body; you're also safeguarding your teeth.

So, remember to prioritize fluoridated water in your daily hydration routine. It's a simple yet effective step towards preserving your smile and promoting overall well-being. Cheers to a hydrated and happy you!

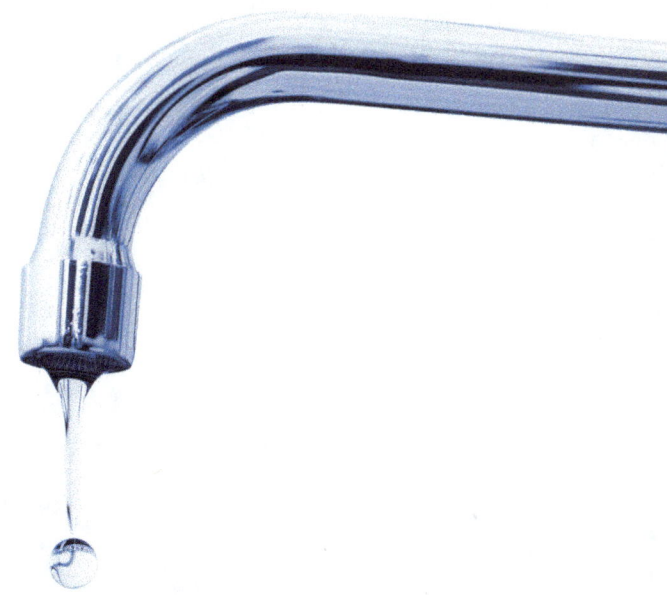

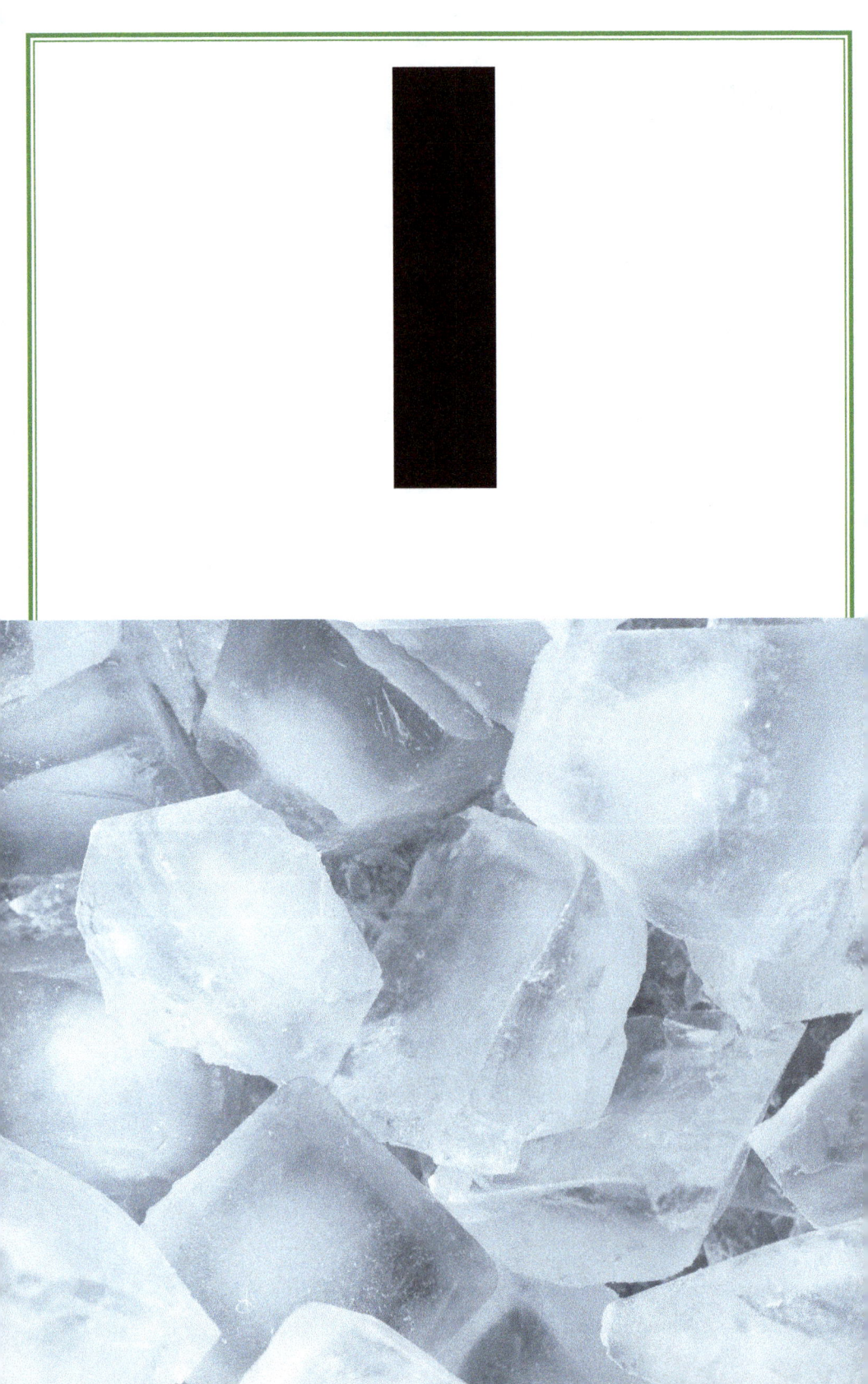

ICE

Ice, Ice, Baby

The Cool Truth About Ice and Your Teeth:
Ice: it's the perfect partner for a refreshing drink, the savior of a scorching summer day, and for some, an irresistible crunchy treat. But when it comes to the health and whiteness of your teeth, is ice a friend or a foe? Let's chill out and explore the icy facts.

The Temptation of Chewing Ice
I know, I know. Trust me, I know. We've all been there—nursing the last few sips of a cool beverage and suddenly, the ice cubes call out to be crunched. That satisfying crunch is tempting, but before you indulge, it's important to understand what happens to your teeth when you give in to that icy temptation.

Ice and Tooth Enamel: A Rocky Relationship
Your tooth enamel is the hardest substance in your body, but it's not indestructible. Chewing on ice can cause micro-cracks and chips in the enamel. Over time, these tiny fissures can lead to bigger problems:

- **Increased Sensitivity:** Damaged enamel can expose the more sensitive inner layers of your teeth, making them more susceptible to hot, cold, or sweet foods and drinks.
- **Staining and Discoloration:** The cracks and chips in your enamel can make it easier for stains from coffee, wine, and other foods to take hold, dulling your bright smile.
- **Risk of Cavities:** Once your enamel is compromised, your teeth are more vulnerable to decay, leading to cavities that can further darken and damage your smile.

The Whitening Woes
When it comes to whitening, keeping your enamel intact is crucial. Strong, healthy enamel is the foundation of a healthy, white smile.

Here's how ice can impact your efforts:
- **Weakened Enamel:** As mentioned, chewing ice can weaken and damage enamel, which is counterproductive if you're aiming for a whiter, brighter smile. Weak enamel not only stains more easily but also responds less effectively to whitening treatments.

My best advice is to skip the ice.

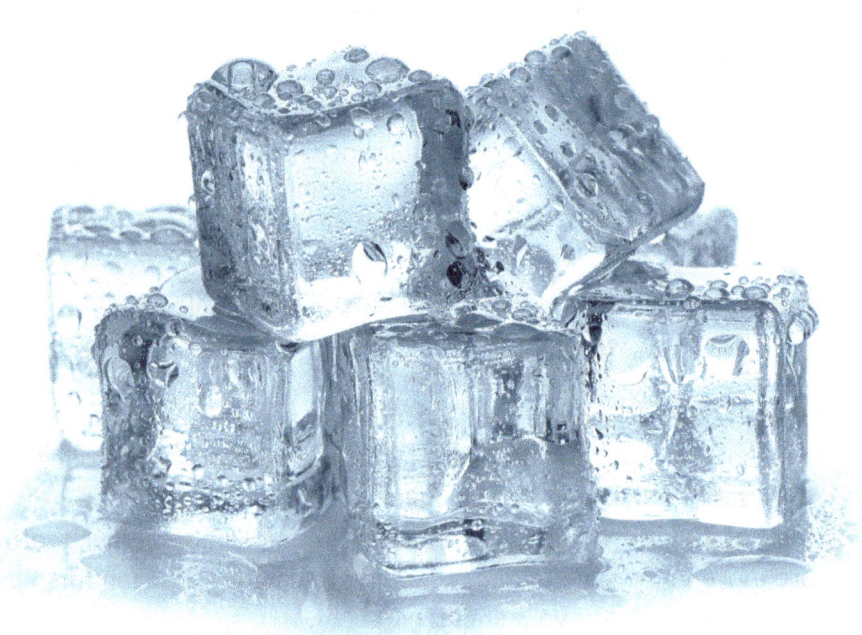

Iron Supplements

Beware of the Dark Side - How these supplements can tarnish your smile.

Traditional oral iron supplements can be a headache for those working to keep their smile white and bright.

Iron, being a metal, has the unfortunate ability to stain teeth on contact. And it's not just iron—metals like silver and manganese can also leave their mark, making it even more important to take precautions.

To keep your smile bright mix your iron dose in water, fruit juice, or tomato juice. Use a drinking straw to help keep the supplement away from your teeth.

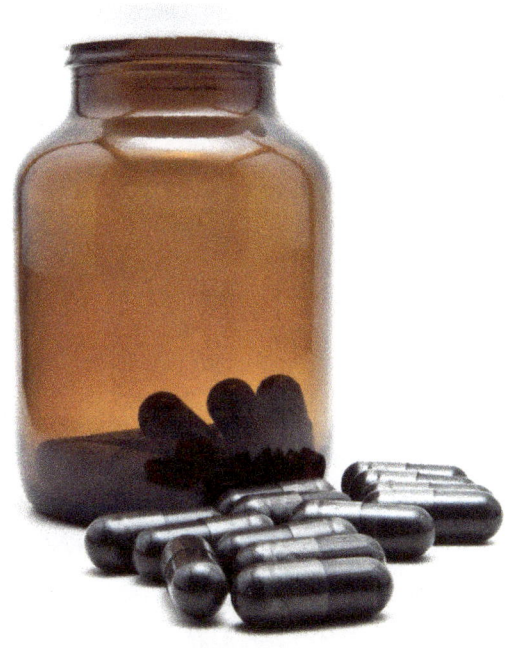

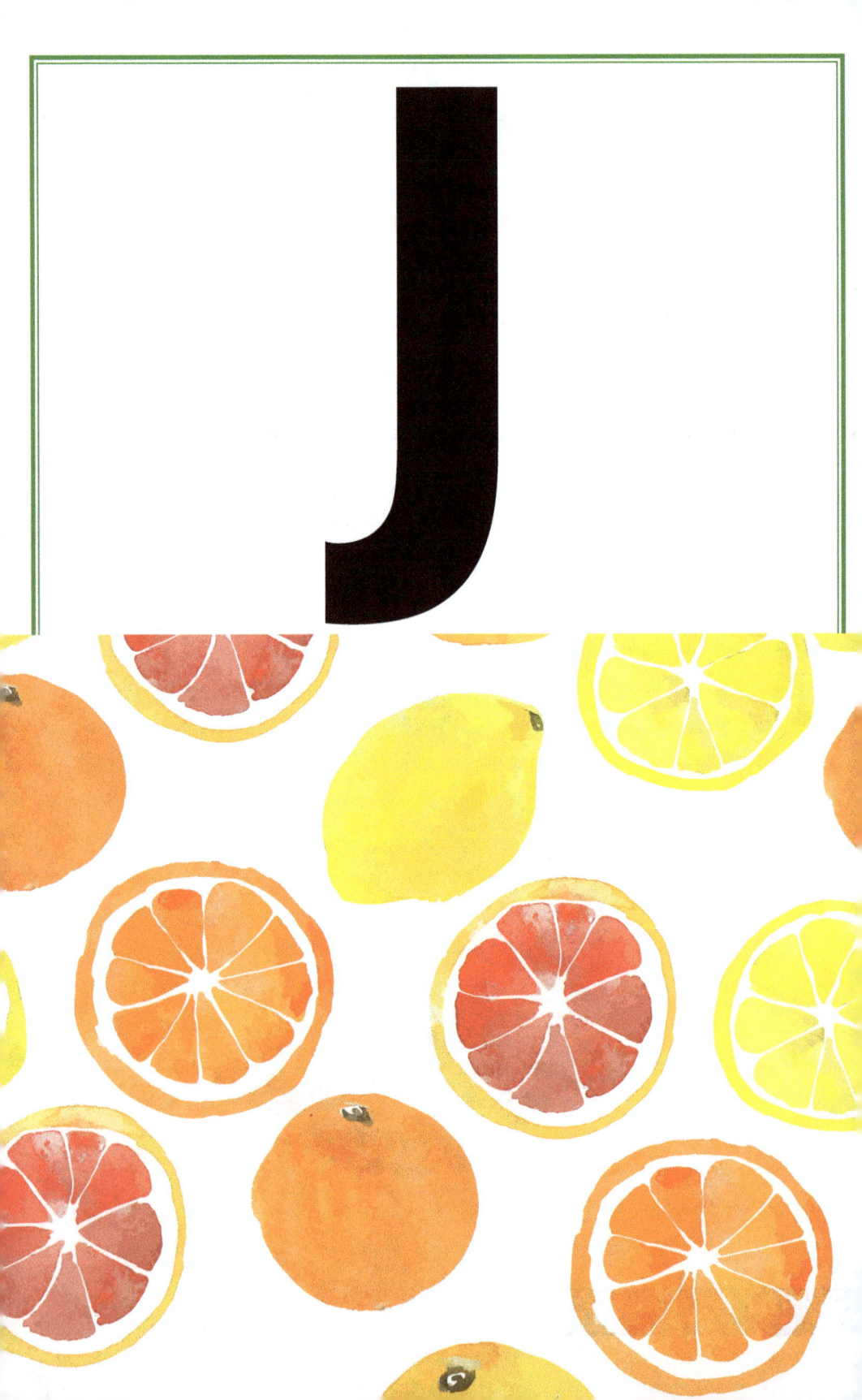

Juice

Protect Your Pearly Whites

Beware of Staining Juices

Grapes, pomegranates, and cranberries boast vibrant colors due to their high pigmentation, but they also pose a risk of staining your teeth.

If you indulge in these fruit juices, take precautions to safeguard your smile.

Consider rinsing your mouth with water immediately afterward, or opt for drinking juices through a straw to minimize direct contact with the front surfaces of your teeth. By incorporating these simple habits into your routine, you can enjoy the benefits of these fruits without compromising your teeth's brightness.

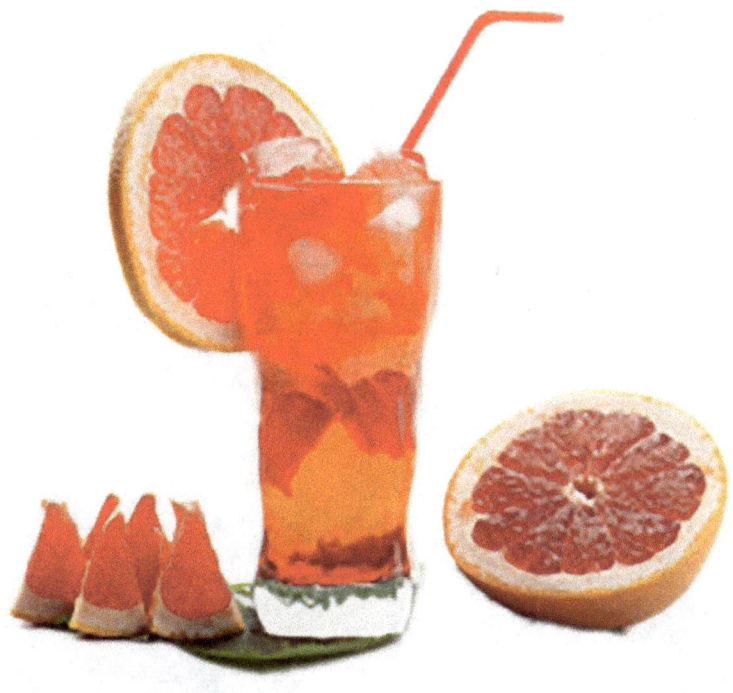

K

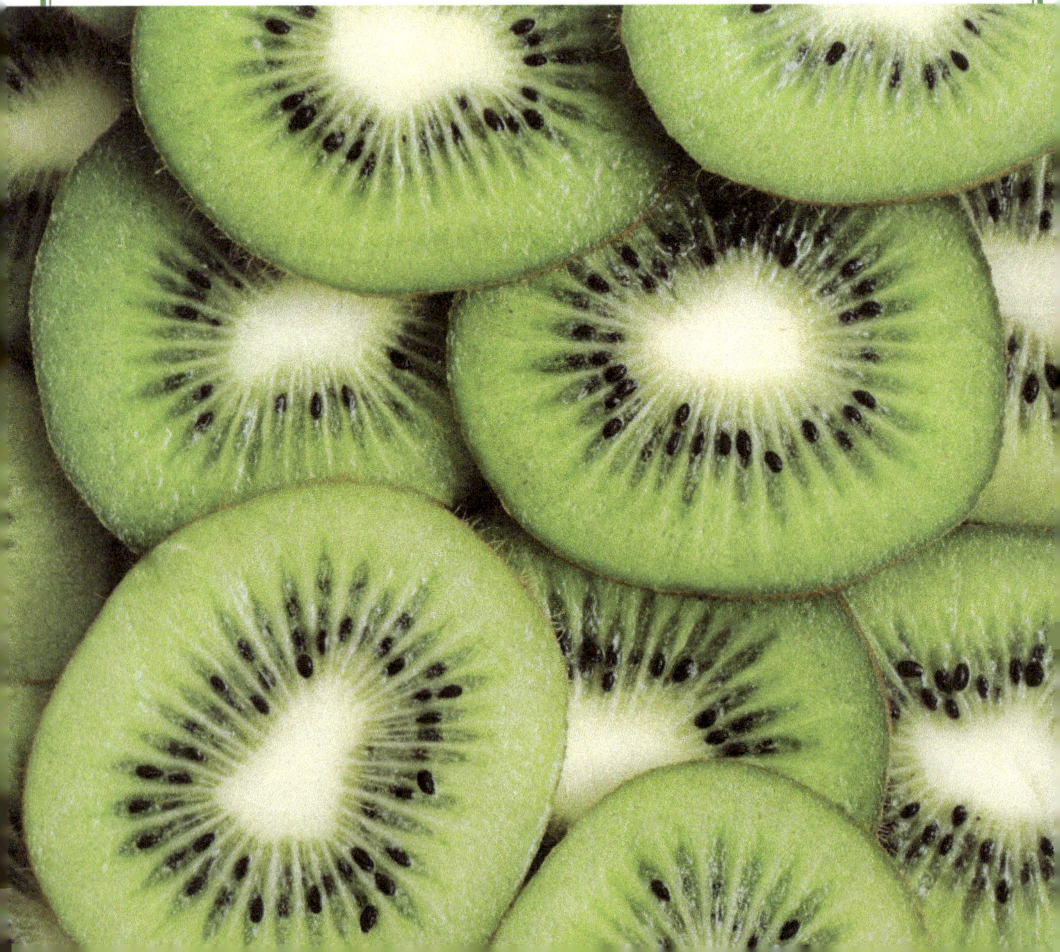

Kale

A Leafy Green for a Brighter Smile

Kale is more than just a nutrient-dense superfood—it's also a natural ally for whitening your teeth. Its high fiber content helps stimulate saliva production, which aids in washing away food particles and reducing plaque buildup. The leafy green is rich in calcium and vitamins that support strong enamel and overall oral health. Additionally, the natural crunchiness of kale helps gently scrub away surface stains, contributing to a cleaner, brighter smile.

Incorporate kale into your diet for a delicious way to enhance your oral care routine and enjoy a naturally whiter, healthier smile!

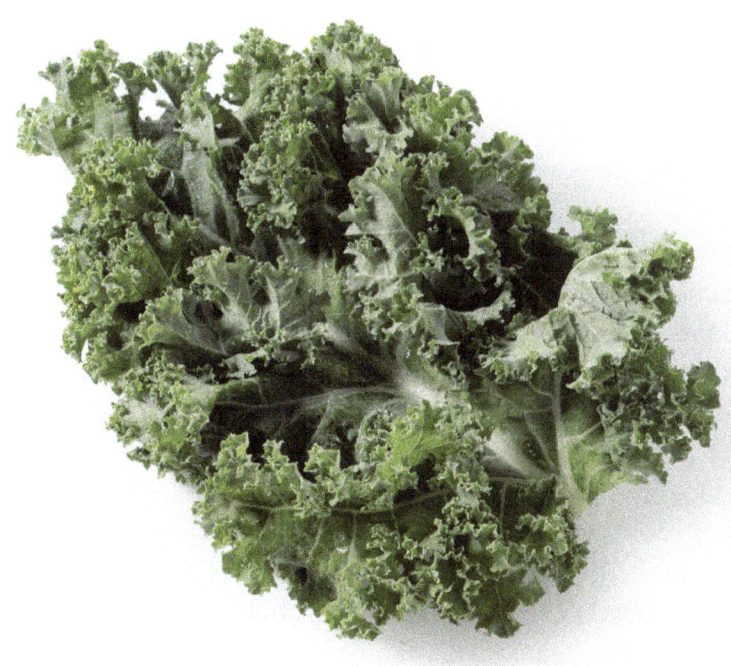

Kiwi

A Delicious Boost for Teeth and Gum Health

Kiwi is a nutrient-rich fruit that offers several benefits for your oral health, including contributing to whiter teeth and healthier gums.

Here's how kiwi can help support your dental health:

1. **Rich in Vitamin C:** Kiwi is packed with vitamin C, which is essential for maintaining healthy gums. Vitamin C helps to strengthen the blood vessels and connective tissues in the gums, reducing the risk of gum inflammation and periodontal disease.
2. **Promotes Collagen Production:** The high vitamin C content in kiwi supports collagen production, which is crucial for maintaining the structural integrity of your gums. This helps keep your gums firm and resilient against infections.
3. **Natural Enzymes for Stain Removal:** Kiwi contains natural enzymes such as actinidin, which can help break down protein-based stains on the teeth, contributing to a brighter smile. These enzymes can gently assist in removing surface stains caused by foods and beverages.
4. **Antioxidant Properties:** The antioxidants found in kiwi, including vitamin C and polyphenols, help protect your oral tissues from oxidative stress and inflammation, promoting overall oral health.
5. **Promotes Saliva Production:** Eating kiwi can stimulate saliva production, which naturally cleanses the mouth by washing away food particles and bacteria. This helps prevent plaque buildup and reduces the risk of cavities.
6. **Fiber Content:** The fiber in kiwi acts as a natural scrub for your teeth, helping to remove debris and stains from the tooth surface as you chew. This gentle scrubbing action contributes to maintaining a cleaner and whiter smile.

Incorporating Kiwi into Your Diet:
- **Fresh and Raw:** Enjoy kiwi fresh and raw to reap the full benefits of its nutrients and enzymes. Slice it into salads, or eat it on its own as a tasty snack.
- **Smoothies:** Add kiwi to your smoothies for a refreshing and nutritious boost. Pair it with other fruits and leafy greens for a healthy blend.
- **Regular Consumption:** Make kiwi a regular part of your diet to continuously benefit from its oral health properties.

While kiwi offers several benefits for your teeth and gums, it is important to maintain a balanced diet and follow a proper oral hygiene routine, including regular brushing, flossing, and dental check-ups, to keep your smile bright and healthy.

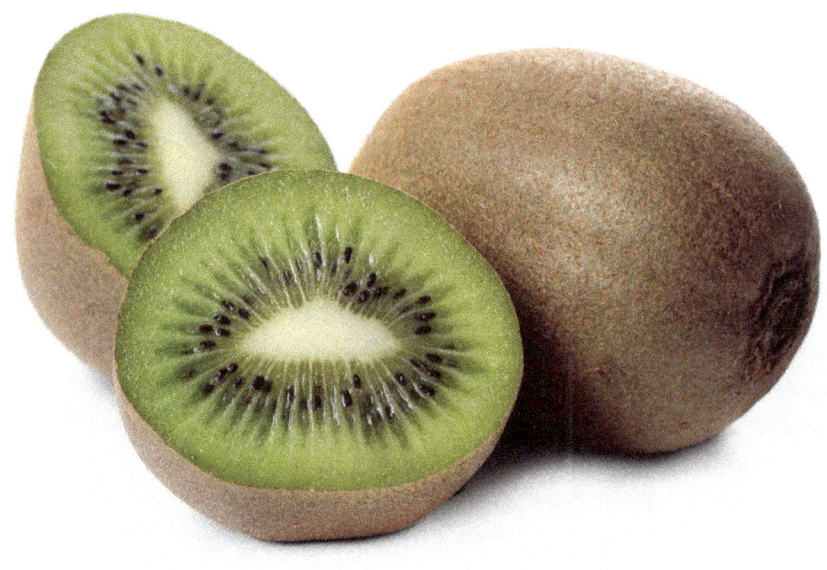

Kombucha

The Fizzy Elixir for a Healthier, Brighter Smile

Kombucha, the trendy fermented tea beverage known for its tangy taste and probiotic benefits, can also play a role in promoting a whiter, brighter, and healthier smile. This effervescent drink is more than just a refreshing treat—it's a natural ally in your oral health journey.

Whitening and Brightening Benefits

Kombucha is rich in organic acids, such as acetic acid and gluconic acid, which can help break down stains on the teeth. These mild acids gently dissolve surface stains, contributing to a brighter smile without the harshness of chemical whiteners. Additionally, the effervescence of kombucha can provide a gentle scrubbing action on the teeth, further aiding in the removal of stains.

Healthier Teeth and Gums

Kombucha offers several benefits that support overall oral health:

1. **Probiotics:** Kombucha is packed with beneficial probiotics that help balance the oral microbiome. A healthy oral microbiome is essential for reducing harmful bacteria that cause cavities, gum disease, and bad breath. By promoting beneficial bacteria, kombucha helps maintain a healthier mouth environment.
2. **Antioxidants:** The tea base of kombucha, often green or black tea, is rich in antioxidants like polyphenols. These antioxidants protect gums and teeth from oxidative stress and inflammation, reducing the risk of gum disease and promoting healthier oral tissues.
3. **Enzymes:** The fermentation process of kombucha produces enzymes that can aid in breaking down food particles in the mouth, helping to prevent plaque buildup and cavities.
4. **Vitamins:** Kombucha contains vitamins like B vitamins and vitamin C, which support healthy gums and help repair oral tissues.

How to Incorporate Kombucha into Your Smile Diet

Incorporate kombucha into your diet as a refreshing beverage. Opt for varieties with minimal added sugars to avoid potential harm to your teeth from excess sugar consumption. Enjoy kombucha as a mid-day refreshment or a replacement for sugary sodas.

Conclusion

Kombucha is not just a health-conscious beverage choice; it also offers benefits that support a whiter, brighter, and healthier smile. By integrating kombucha into your daily routine, you can enjoy its natural advantages while working towards a radiant grin. Let the power of probiotics and antioxidants in kombucha enhance your oral health journey, making your smile shine with confidence.

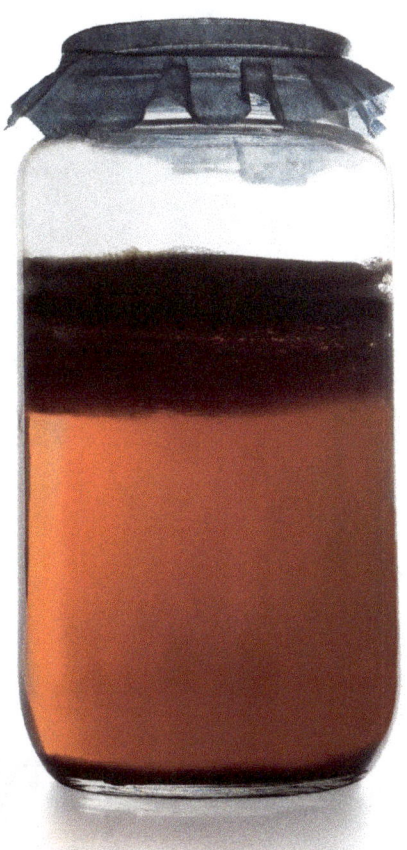

L

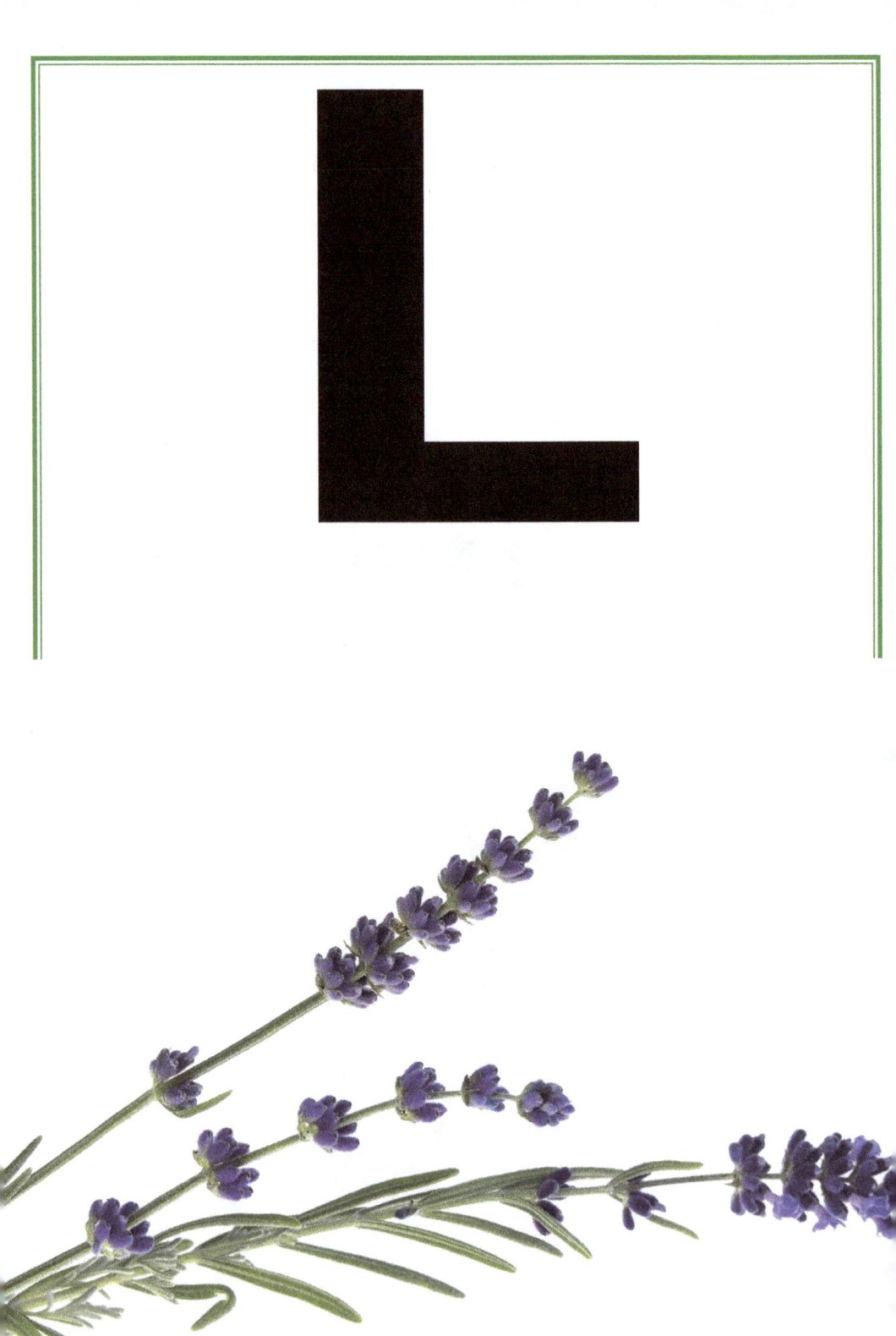

Lavender

The Floral Ally for a Healthier, Brighter Smile

Lavender, renowned for its calming scent and vibrant purple blooms, is more than just a fragrant herb. This versatile plant offers unique benefits for oral health, helping to whiten, brighten, and maintain a healthy smile.

Whitening and Brightening Benefits
Lavender contains natural compounds with mild abrasive properties that can help polish teeth and remove surface stains, contributing to a brighter smile. While not a direct teeth whitener, lavender's cleansing action can complement your oral care routine by promoting a cleaner, more radiant appearance.

Healthier Teeth and Gums
Lavender offers several benefits that support overall oral health:

1. **Antimicrobial Properties:** Lavender is known for its antimicrobial and antibacterial effects, which can help reduce harmful bacteria in the mouth. This property aids in preventing cavities, reducing plaque buildup, and promoting fresher breath.
2. **Anti-Inflammatory Effects:** The anti-inflammatory compounds in lavender, such as linalool and linalyl acetate, can help soothe irritated gums and reduce inflammation. This is beneficial for preventing gum disease and maintaining healthy gum tissues.
3. **Antioxidants:** Lavender is rich in antioxidants that protect oral tissues from oxidative stress and damage, promoting healthier gums and teeth.
4. **Aromatic Benefits:** The pleasant aroma of lavender can contribute to fresh breath, making it a natural choice for mouth rinses and dental products.

How to Incorporate Lavender into Your Smile Diet
Lavender can be used in several ways to support oral health:

- **Lavender Tea:** Drinking lavender tea can provide soothing benefits for the mouth and promote relaxation.
- **Mouth Rinse:** Use diluted lavender essential oil in a homemade mouth rinse to harness its antimicrobial and aromatic properties. Always ensure essential oils are properly diluted before use.
- **Lavender Infused Toothpaste:** Look for toothpaste or dental products containing lavender extract for added benefits in your oral care routine.

Conclusion
Lavender is more than a fragrant flower; it is a powerful ally in maintaining a whiter, brighter, and healthier smile. By incorporating lavender into your daily routine, you can enjoy its natural benefits while promoting oral health and confidence. Let the soothing power of lavender enhance your journey to a radiant smile, transforming your oral care with its floral charm.

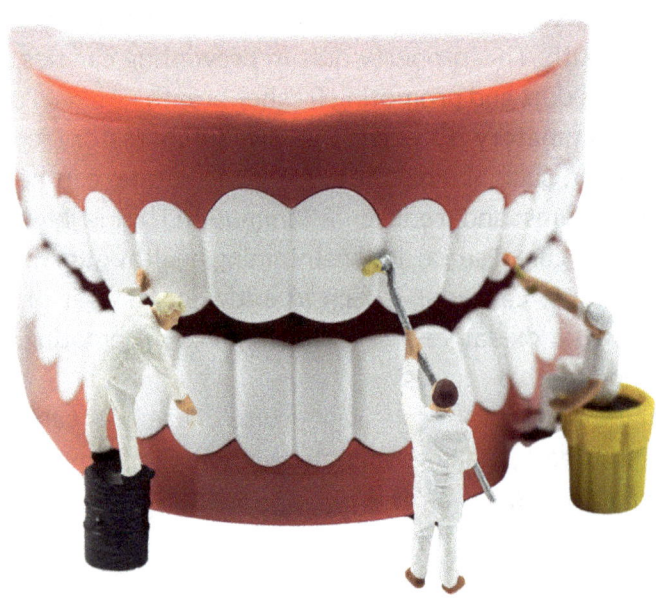

Leafy Greens

The Unsung Heroes Behind Every Radiant Smile

Include leafy greens such as spinach and kale in your diet for optimal oral health, as advised in **The Smile Diet** Book. Their high calcium content supports enamel strength, contributing to a whiter smile.

Elevate your smile with the power of greens! Dive into **The Smile Diet** Book to uncover how leafy greens like spinach and kale, packed with vitamins and minerals, contribute to optimal oral health and a dazzling white smile.

Grab-and-go veggies like green beans, broccoli, celery, and carrots are great for your smile. These crunchy snacks stimulate saliva, helping prevent plaque buildup and whitening your teeth. Plus, biting into them and chewing gently scrubs your teeth, lifting surface stains for a whiter, brighter and healthier smile.

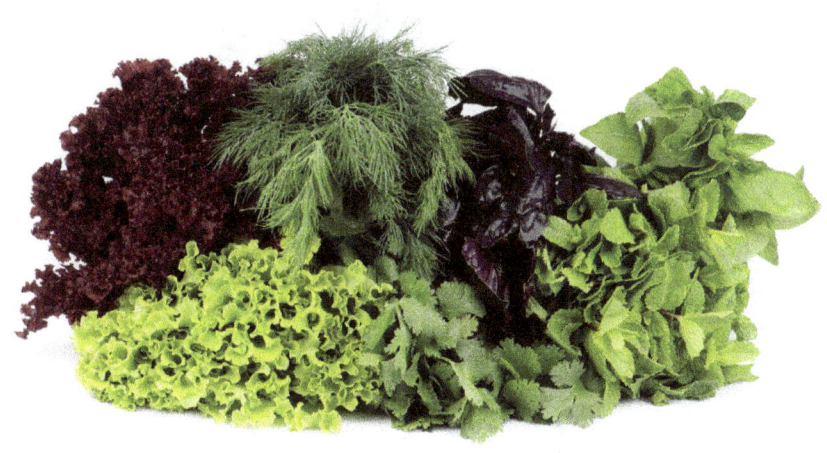

Lettuce

A Crisp Choice for a Brighter Smile

Lettuce isn't just a staple for your salads—it's also a natural helper for whitening your teeth. Its high water content and crisp texture promote saliva production, which assists in washing away food particles and reducing plaque buildup. Lettuce is rich in vitamins and minerals that support overall oral health and strengthen enamel, contributing to a naturally brighter smile. Enjoy this refreshing leafy green in your meals to boost your oral care routine and help maintain a cleaner, whiter smile effortlessly!

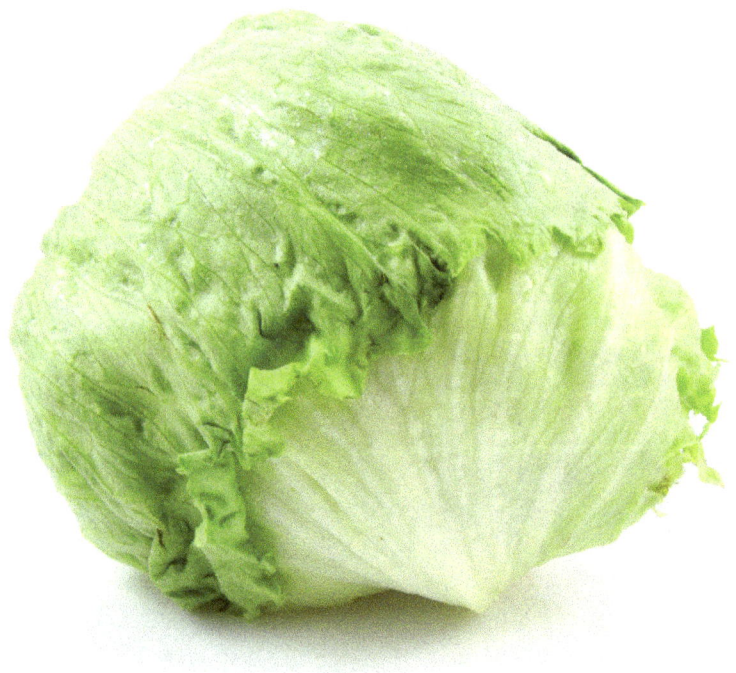

Limes

A Zesty Boost for a Brighter Smile

Limes are not just a tangy addition to your dishes—they can also help naturally whiten your teeth. Rich in vitamin C and citric acid, limes support gum health and aid in breaking down surface stains. Their natural acidity helps to dissolve discoloration, while the vitamin C promotes strong enamel and overall oral health.

However, it's important to use limes in moderation and rinse your mouth with water afterward to protect your enamel from excessive acid exposure. Enjoy this citrus fruit as a zesty ingredient in your diet and let its natural properties contribute to a brighter, healthier smile!

Grab-and-go veggies like green beans, broccoli, celery, and carrots are great for your smile. These crunchy snacks stimulate saliva, helping prevent plaque buildup and whitening your teeth. Plus, biting into them and chewing gently scrubs your teeth, lifting surface stains for a whiter, brighter and healthier smile.

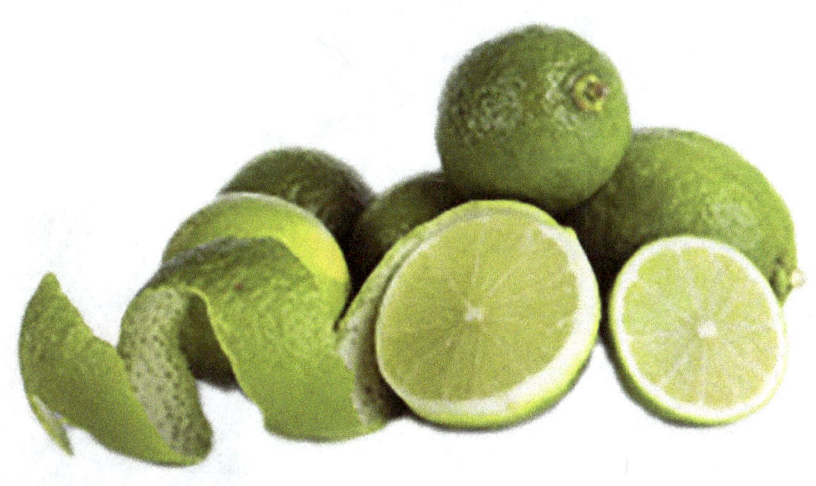

M

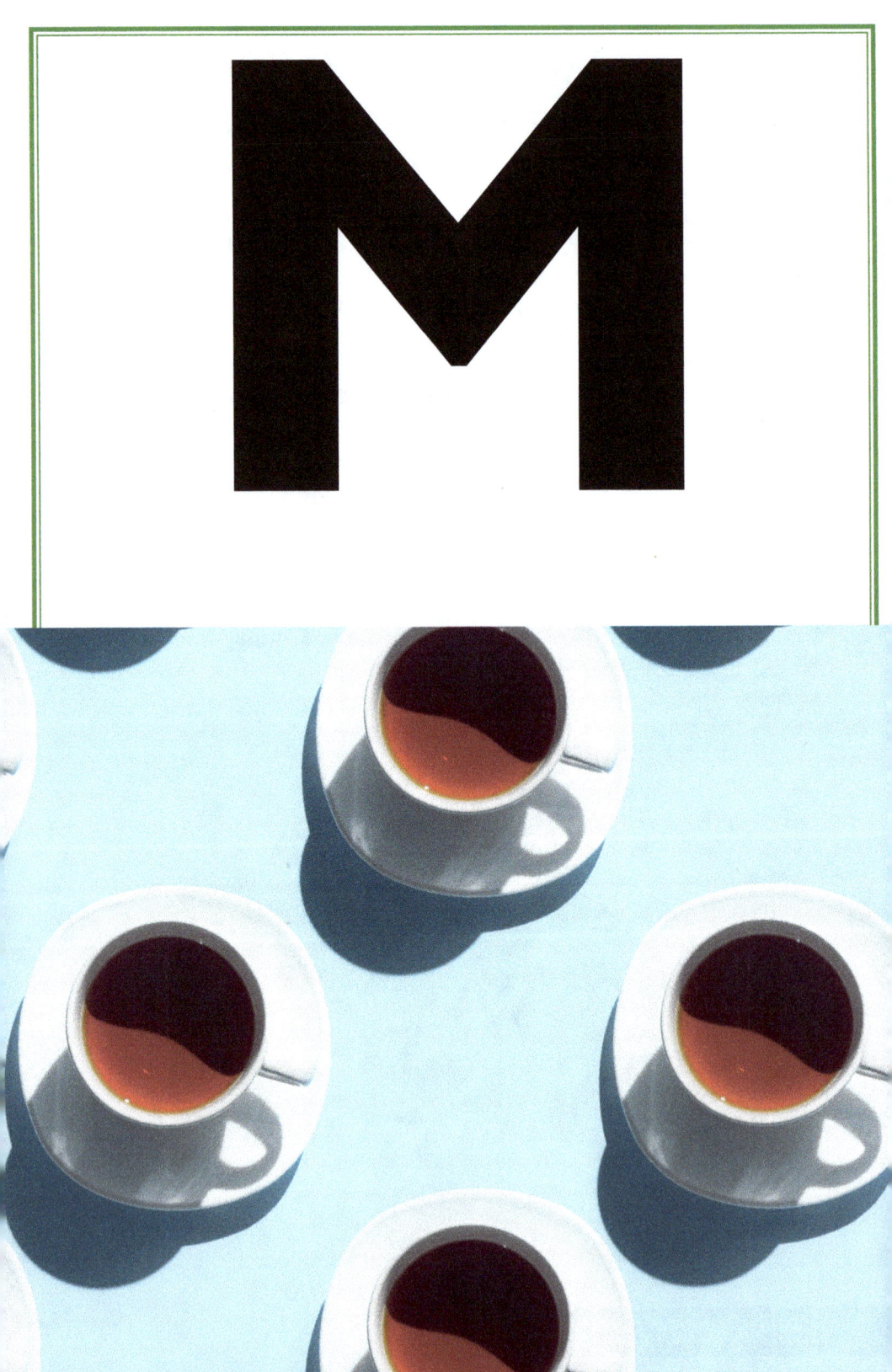

Matcha

A Green Boost for Oral Health and Teeth Whitening

Matcha, a finely ground powder of specially grown and processed green tea leaves, is not only celebrated for its unique flavor and health benefits but also for its potential to enhance oral health and support teeth whitening. Here's how incorporating matcha into your diet can benefit your teeth and gums:

1. **Rich in Antioxidants:** Matcha is packed with antioxidants, particularly catechins like epigallocatechin gallate (EGCG), which help fight bacteria and reduce inflammation in the mouth. These antioxidants can inhibit the growth of harmful bacteria, reducing the risk of cavities and gum disease.
2. **Natural Stain Prevention:** The high levels of catechins in matcha help prevent the formation of plaque and reduce the adherence of bacteria to your teeth, potentially lowering the risk of stains and discoloration. This can contribute to a whiter, brighter smile.
3. **Promotes Healthy Gums:** Matcha contains anti- inflammatory properties that can help soothe and protect gums. By reducing inflammation and bacterial growth, matcha may contribute to healthier gums and lower the risk of gingivitis and periodontal disease.
4. **Neutralizes Acid:** Matcha can help neutralize acids in the mouth that erode tooth enamel and lead to decay. By maintaining a more balanced pH level, matcha supports the health and integrity of your teeth.
5. **Freshens Breath:** The natural compounds in matcha have deodorizing properties that can help freshen breath by reducing the presence of odor-causing bacteria in the mouth.

Incorporating Matcha into Your Routine:

- **Matcha Tea:** Enjoy a cup of matcha tea as a refreshing and healthy alternative to sugary beverages that can contribute to tooth decay.
- **Smoothies:** Add matcha powder to your favorite smoothie for a nutrient-rich boost that benefits your oral health.
- **Baking and Cooking:** Incorporate matcha into recipes for baked goods, oatmeal, or yogurt for a flavorful twist and added health benefits.

While matcha offers numerous oral health benefits, it is important to maintain good oral hygiene practices, including regular brushing and flossing, to achieve and maintain a healthy, white smile.

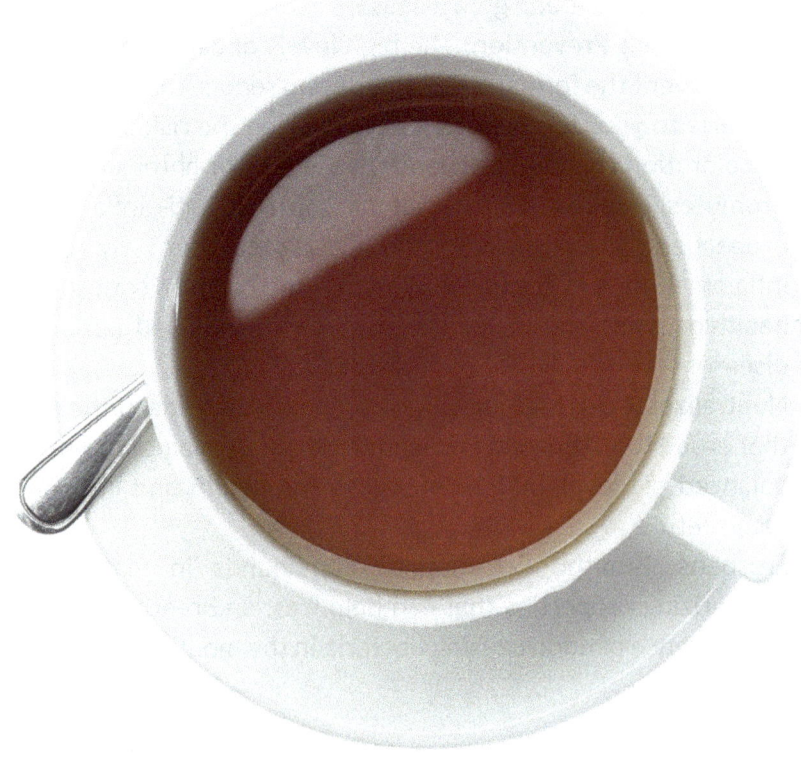

Medications That Can Stain Teeth

Watch Out for These Smile Saboteurs!

Certain medications have the potential to cause tooth discoloration. For example, the antibiotic tetracycline can lead to gray teeth in children whose teeth are still developing. Antibacterial mouthwashes containing chlorhexidine or cetylpyridinium chloride can also contribute to staining. Additionally, some antihistamines, antipsychotic drugs, blood pressure medications, iron supplements, and excessive fluoride can cause teeth to become discolored. If teeth whitening treatments don't provide the desired results, consider discussing dental bonding with your dentist. This procedure involves applying a tooth-colored material to improve the appearance of stained teeth.

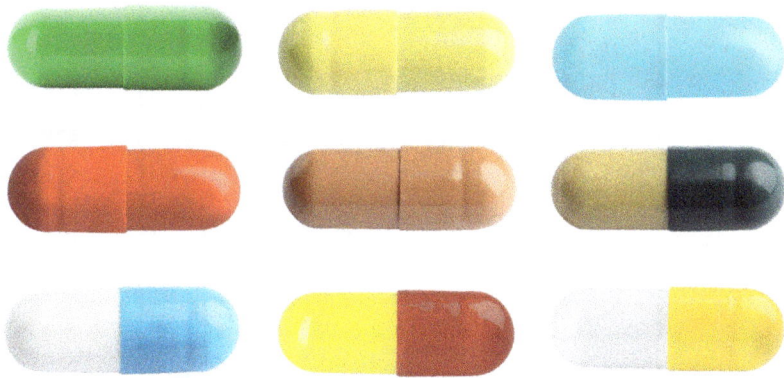

Got Milk?

How about a white smile?
Exploring the Milky Way to Whiter Teeth!

Milk is not only a nutritious drink but also a natural aid for whitening your teeth. Rich in calcium and phosphorus, milk supports strong enamel and helps remineralize your teeth, which can prevent and reduce staining. The proteins in milk form a protective layer on your teeth, which can shield them from acids and stains. Additionally, milk's high water content helps wash away food particles and bacteria. Incorporate this creamy beverage into your diet to enhance your oral health and promote a naturally whiter, healthier smile!

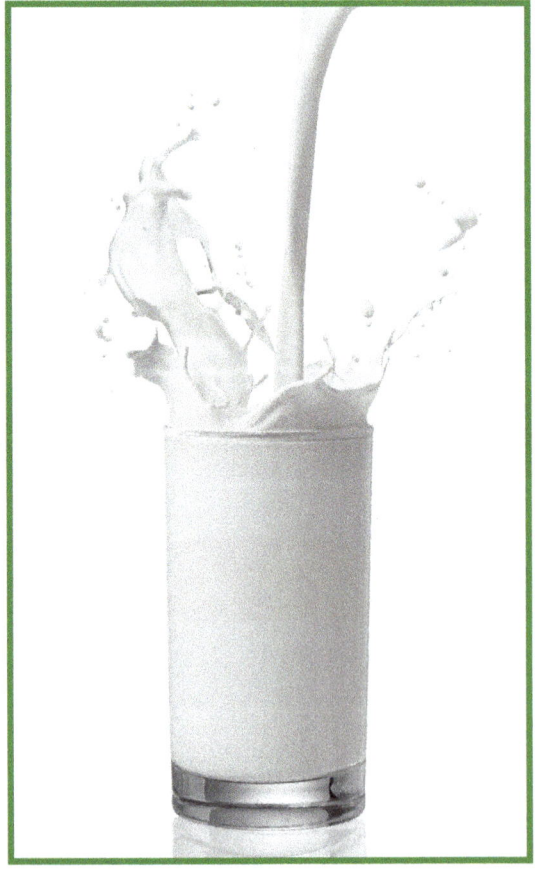

Miso

A Fermented Powerhouse for Oral Health

Miso, a traditional Japanese fermented soybean paste, is not only a flavorful addition to soups and sauces but also offers several benefits for your teeth and gums. Here's how incorporating miso into your diet can contribute to a healthier, whiter smile:

1. **Rich in Probiotics:** Miso contains probiotics, which are beneficial bacteria that help maintain a healthy balance of microorganisms in your mouth. This can reduce harmful bacteria that contribute to tooth decay and gum disease.
2. **Promotes Oral Health:** The probiotics in miso can help decrease oral inflammation and improve gum health by supporting a balanced oral microbiome. A healthy microbiome reduces the risk of periodontal disease and keeps gums strong.
3. **Calcium and Phosphorus Content:** Miso is a source of calcium and phosphorus, essential minerals for maintaining strong teeth and supporting enamel remineralization. These minerals help prevent tooth decay and keep your teeth healthy.
4. **Antioxidant Properties:** The fermentation process of miso results in the production of antioxidants, which help protect oral tissues from oxidative stress and reduce inflammation in the gums.
5. **Enzyme-Rich:** Miso contains enzymes that can aid in breaking down food particles, potentially reducing the risk of plaque buildup. Less plaque means a lower risk of stains and cavities.
6. **Stimulates Saliva Production:** Eating miso-based dishes can help stimulate saliva production, which naturally cleanses the mouth by washing away food particles and neutralizing acids that erode enamel.

Incorporating Miso into Your Diet:

- **Miso Soup:** Enjoy miso soup as a comforting and nutritious starter or snack. It's a simple way to incorporate miso into your daily routine.
- **Marinades and Dressings:** Use miso as a base for marinades and salad dressings to add a rich, umami flavor while benefiting your oral health.
- **Fermented Foods:** Pair miso with other fermented foods like sauerkraut or kimchi for an added boost to your oral microbiome.

While miso offers several benefits for your oral health, it is important to maintain a balanced diet and follow a proper oral hygiene routine, including regular brushing, flossing, and dental check-ups, to keep your smile bright and healthy.

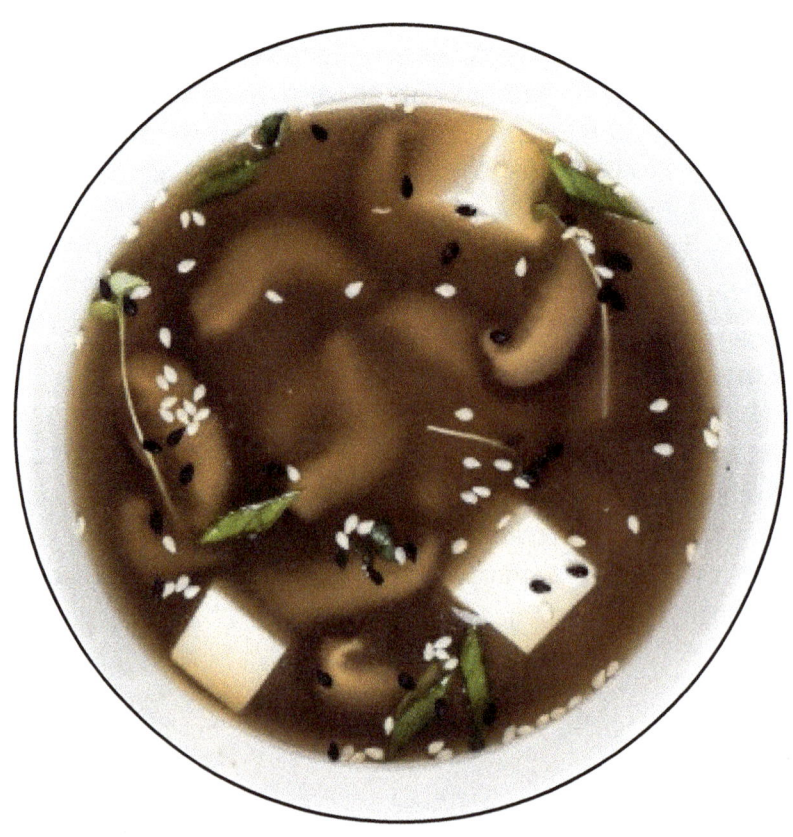

Mint Leaves

A Fresh Boost for a Brighter Smile

Mint leaves are more than just a refreshing herb—they offer natural benefits for whitening your teeth. Their natural oils have antibacterial properties that help combat plaque and freshen breath, while their mild abrasiveness can gently remove surface stains.

Mint's cooling effect also promotes saliva production, which aids in washing away food particles and bacteria that can lead to discoloration. Incorporate mint leaves into your diet or use them in homemade mouth rinses to enjoy a fresher, cleaner smile and enhance your oral care routine naturally!

The Freshness Factor
Whether you're feeling drained after a social event or surviving a loooooong, boring meeting, popping a mint leaf, or enjoying a sugarfree mint can instantly refresh you. It'll not only give you a burst of energy to put some ZZZIP back in your step but also help banish that lingering stale coffee breath.

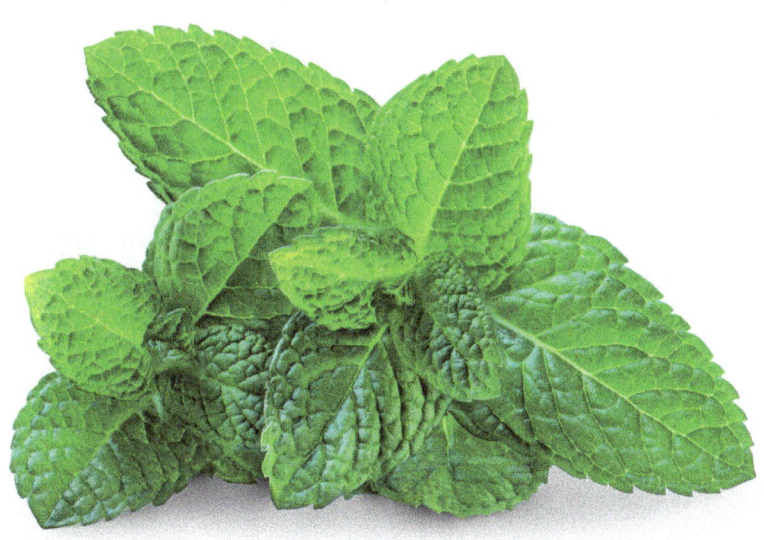

Melons

A Refreshing Boost for Oral Health

Melons, such as cantaloupe, honeydew, and watermelon, are not only refreshing and hydrating but also offer several benefits for your teeth and gums. Here's how incorporating melons into your diet can contribute to a healthier, brighter smile:

1. **High Water Content:** Melons have a high water content, which helps stimulate saliva production. Saliva plays a crucial role in naturally cleansing the mouth, washing away food particles, and neutralizing acids that can erode tooth enamel.
2. **Rich in Vitamins:** Melons are rich in vitamins A and C, which are essential for maintaining healthy gums and oral tissues. Vitamin C, in particular, helps strengthen blood vessels and connective tissues in the gums, reducing the risk of gum disease.
3. **Antioxidant Properties:** The antioxidants found in melons, such as beta-carotene, help protect oral tissues from oxidative stress and inflammation, contributing to overall oral health.
4. **Low in Acid:** Melons have a low acidity level, making them a toothfriendly fruit option. Consuming low-acid foods helps protect tooth enamel from erosion and reduces the risk of enamel wear.
5. **Fiber Content:** The fiber in melons helps promote oral health by gently scrubbing the teeth as you chew, which can aid in removing surface stains and reducing plaque buildup.
6. **Hydration:** Staying hydrated is essential for maintaining good oral health. The high water content in melons helps keep you hydrated, which supports saliva production and overall oral health.

Incorporating Melons into Your Diet:

- **Snacks and Salads:** Enjoy fresh slices of melon as a healthy snack or add them to fruit salads for a refreshing treat.
- **Smoothies:** Blend melons into smoothies for a hydrating and nutritious beverage that supports your oral health.

- **Desserts:** Use melons as a base for light, refreshing desserts that are both tooth-friendly and delicious.

While melons offer several benefits for your oral health, it is important to maintain a balanced diet and follow a proper oral hygiene routine, including regular brushing, flossing, and dental check-ups, to keep your smile bright and healthy.

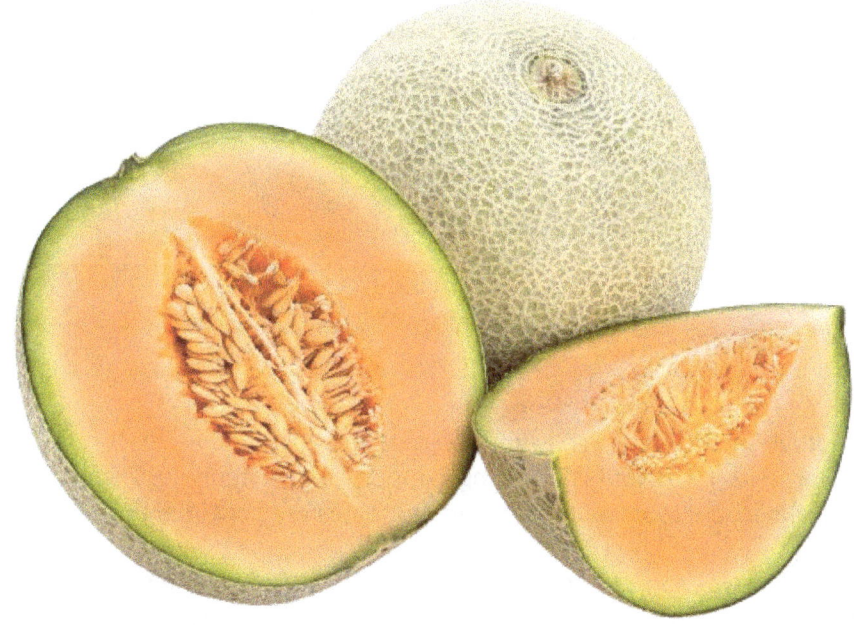

Mushrooms

Can Be Magic for Your Teeth

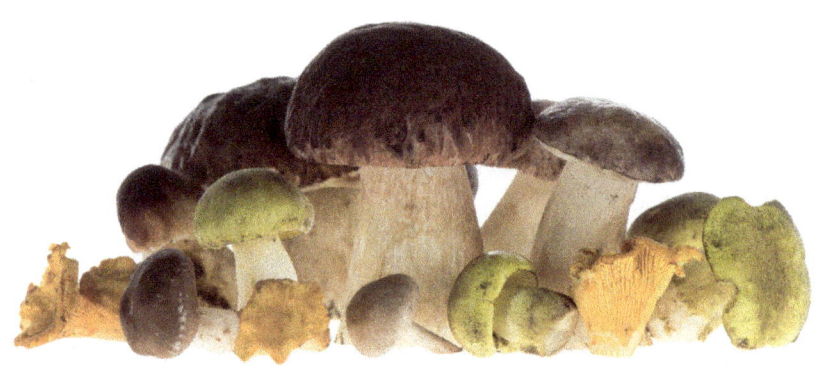

Fungi Fun: Unveiling the Smile-Boosting Benefits of Mushrooms!
Indulge in the delectable goodness of mushrooms, a treasure trove of essential nutrients including copper, zinc, Vitamin B5, selenium, riboflavin, and potassium, crucial for maintaining optimal bone health.

While all edible mushroom varieties contribute to bone strength, it's the remarkable shiitake mushrooms that boast a special ability to enhance dental brilliance. This is owed to their unique component, lentinan, a polysaccharide renowned for its cancer-fighting properties and its ability to combat cavity-causing bacteria within the mouth.

Extensive research has researched the profound effects of shiitake mushrooms on oral health, employing models that closely replicate cariogenic conditions in real life.

The findings revealed that when exposed to shiitake mushroom extract and its sub-fractions, a notable inhibition of dentin demineralization was observed, alongside significant microbial shifts conducive to oral wellbeing.

In their comprehensive study, the researchers emphasized the potent anticarcinogenic potential inherent in shiitake mushrooms, highlighting their ability to safeguard dental health effectively.

Embrace the power of shiitake mushrooms, not just for their exquisite flavor, but for their remarkable contribution to a radiant smile and robust oral hygiene. Shiitake—nature's secret weapon for white, healthy teeth.

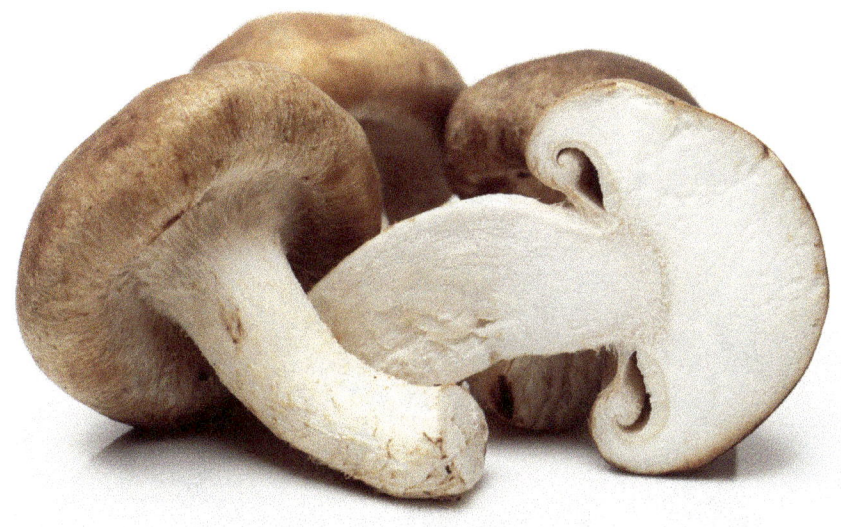

N

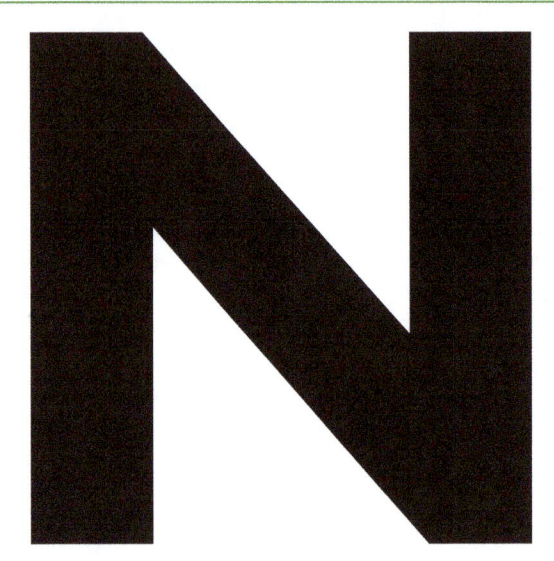

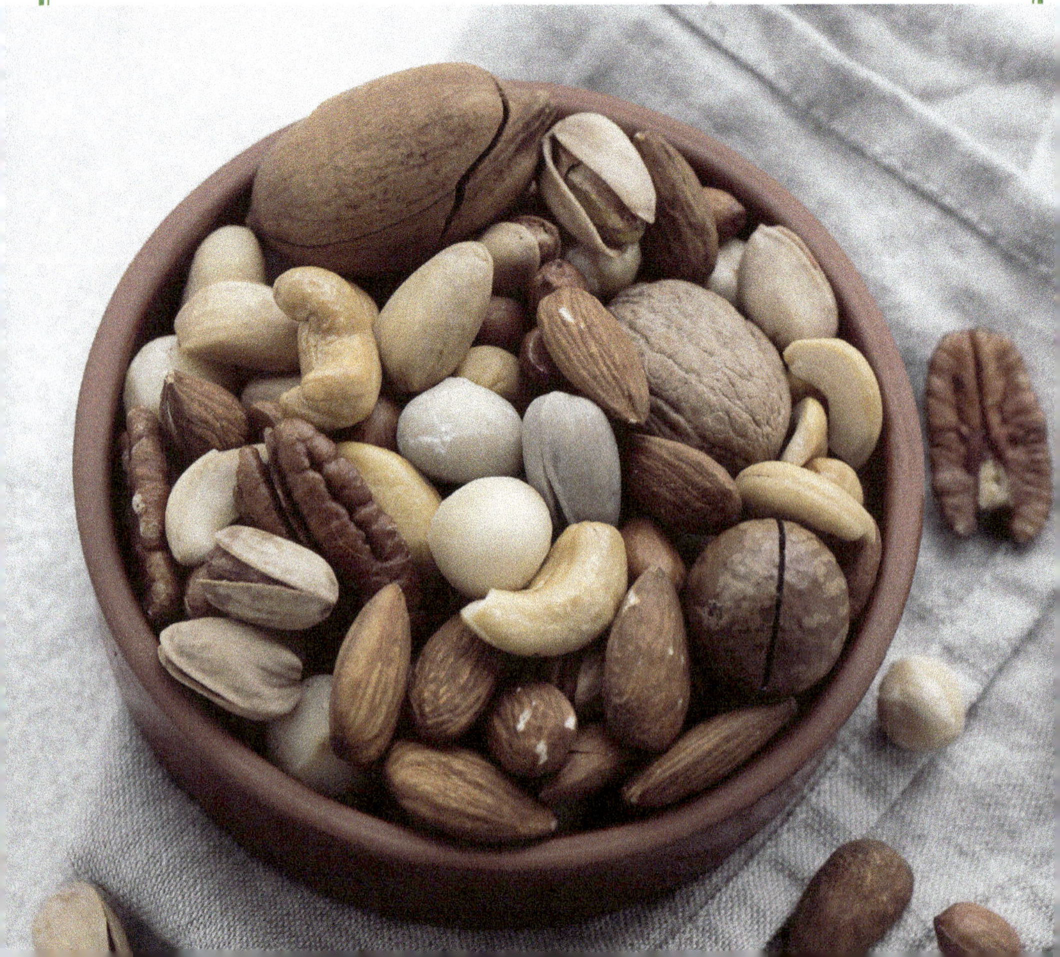

Nectarines

A Sweet Boost for Oral Health

Nectarines, with their juicy and delicious flavor, are not only a delightful summer treat but also offer several benefits for your teeth and gums. Here's how adding nectarines to your diet can contribute to a healthier, whiter smile:

1. **Rich in Vitamins and Minerals:** Nectarines are a good source of vitamins A and C, which are essential for maintaining healthy gums and oral tissues. Vitamin C helps strengthen blood vessels and connective tissues in the gums, reducing the risk of gum disease. Vitamin A supports the production of saliva, which is important for washing away food particles and bacteria.
2. **Hydration and Saliva Production:** The high water content in nectarines helps keep you hydrated, promoting saliva production. Saliva plays a crucial role in neutralizing acids in the mouth, cleansing teeth, and preventing tooth decay.
3. **Antioxidant Properties:** Nectarines contain antioxidants such as beta-carotene and polyphenols, which help protect oral tissues from oxidative stress and inflammation. These antioxidants support overall oral health and can contribute to a brighter smile by reducing the impact of staining and gum issues.
4. **Low in Acid:** Nectarines have a relatively low acidity level compared to other fruits, making them less likely to erode tooth enamel. Consuming low-acid foods helps protect your teeth from enamel wear and keeps them looking whiter.
5. **Natural Fiber:** The natural fiber in nectarines acts like a gentle scrub for your teeth, helping to remove surface stains and plaque buildup as you chew. This can contribute to maintaining a clean and bright smile.

Incorporating Nectarines into Your Diet:
- **Snacks and Desserts:** Enjoy nectarines as a healthy snack or add them to desserts for a sweet, tooth-friendly treat.
- **Smoothies and Salads:** Blend nectarines into smoothies or toss them into salads for a burst of flavor and nutrients that support your oral health.
- **Breakfast:** Add sliced nectarines to your yogurt or cereal for a delicious and nutritious start to your day.

While nectarines offer several benefits for your oral health, it is important to maintain a balanced diet and practice good oral hygiene, including regular brushing, flossing, and dental check-ups, to keep your smile bright and healthy.

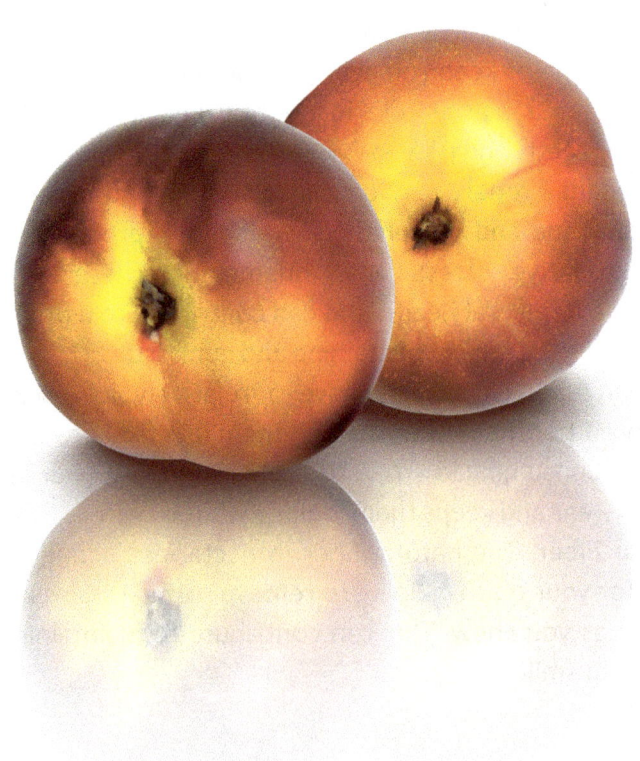

Neem

The Village Pharmacy for a Whiter Smile

Neem, affectionately known as the "village pharmacy," has been a cornerstone of traditional Indian medicine for centuries. Renowned for its antibacterial properties, neem is highly effective in preventing plaque formation and tooth decay. Research published in the Indian Journal of Dental Research supports neem's powerful role in maintaining oral health and whitening teeth.

How to Use Neem for Teeth Whitening
1. **Fresh Neem Leaves:** Chew on fresh neem leaves.
2. **Neem Sticks:** Use neem sticks as a organic toothbrush.
3. **Neem-Based Toothpaste:** Look for neem-based toothpaste available in health stores.

Incorporating neem into your oral care routine can naturally help keep your teeth clean and white. Embrace the age-old wisdom of neem for a healthier, brighter smile.

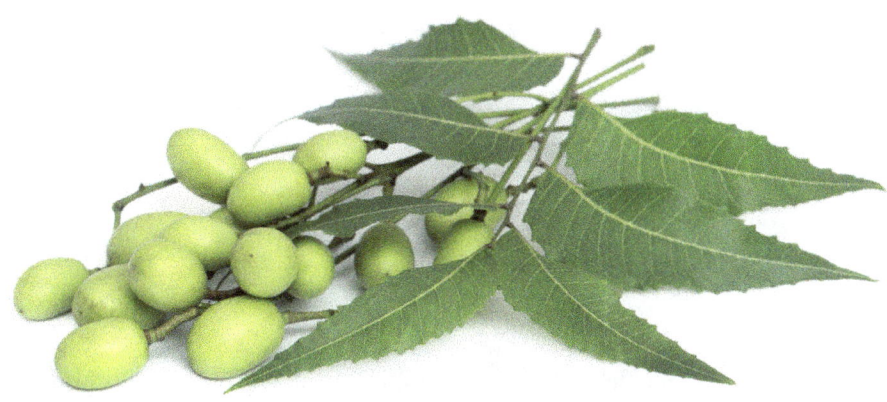

Nuts

Cracking Smiles, One Shell at a Time!

Crack a Smile: Unveiling the Nutty Secrets for Whiter Teeth!

In addition to being a nutritious snack, almonds offer another benefit for your oral health. The ridged edges of almonds provide a gentle abrasive action as you chew, effectively rubbing against your teeth and assisting in the removal of plaque and stains. Embrace the dual benefits of nuts as a satisfying snack and a natural way to maintain a radiant smile.

Nibble Knowledge

Nibble on raw, crunchy almonds as a snack to promote saliva production and help remove surface stains. Almond's texture provides a gentle scrubbing action for whiter teeth.

TIP: A portion of almonds is about 17 nuts, roughly 200 calories per handful. It's easy to go nuts with them, so keep an eye on your portions. Add them to your diet in fun ways, but remember—those tiny nuts can pack a big caloric punch while they are also whitening your teeth!

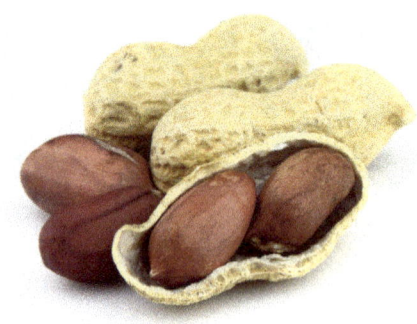

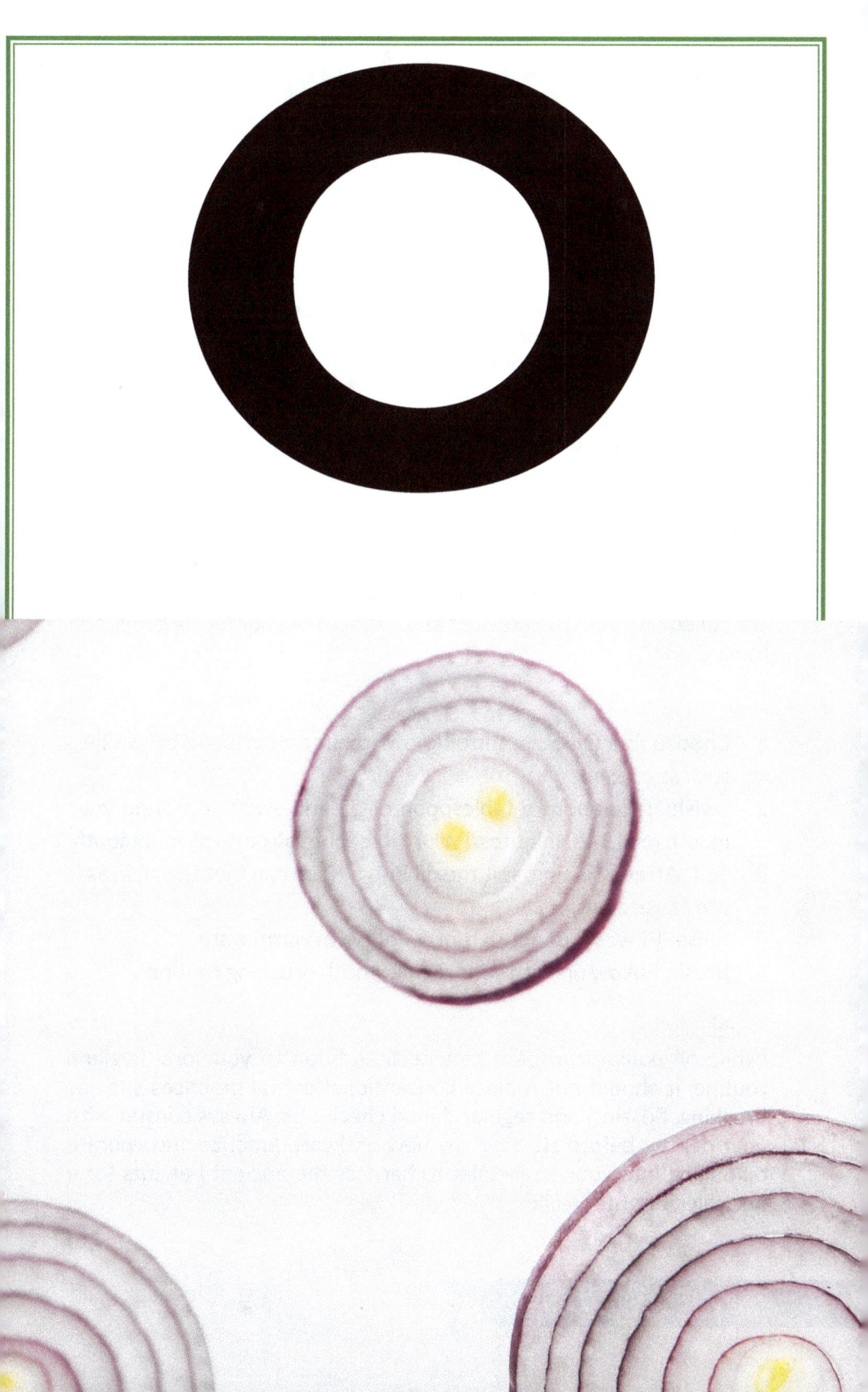

Oil Pulling

Swish and Shine

Oil pulling is an ancient Ayurvedic dental technique that involves swishing oil, typically coconut, sesame, or sunflower oil, in your mouth for about 15-20 minutes. This practice is believed to draw out toxins, reduce harmful bacteria, and improve overall oral hygiene.

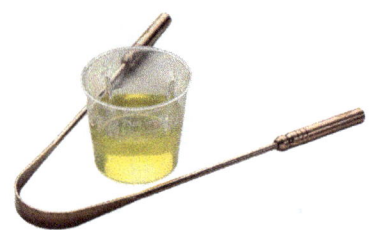

How It Works
The process of oil pulling is simple yet effective. By swishing oil around your mouth, it adheres to the lipid layer of bacteria and other harmful particles. As you continue to swish, these unwanted elements are pulled out from the crevices and surfaces of your teeth, gums, and tongue.

How to Do Oil Pulling
1. **Choose Your Oil:** Select an oil known for its antibacterial properties, such as coconut oil.
2. **Swish:** Take about a tablespoon of oil and swish it around your mouth for 15-20 minutes. Ensure it reaches all parts of your mouth.
3. **Spit:** After swishing, spit the oil into a trash can (not the sink, as it can cause clogs).
4. **Rinse:** Rinse your mouth thoroughly with warm water.
5. **Brush:** Follow up with your regular tooth brushing routine.

Things to Consider
While oil pulling can be a beneficial addition to your oral hygiene routine, it should not replace conventional dental practices such as brushing, flossing, and regular dental check-ups. Always consult with your dentist before starting any new oral care practice. Incorporate oil pulling into your Smile Diet to harness the ancient benefits for a healthier, brighter smile!

Coconut Oil Pulling: A Natural Remedy for Whiter Teeth

If you've explored natural dental remedies, you've likely come across "oil pulling." This practice involves swishing edible oil, usually coconut oil, around your mouth to improve dental health and whiten your teeth.

Why Coconut Oil?

Coconut oil is preferred for oil pulling because it benefits your gums, removes plaque, reduces your risk of bad breath, and also has teeth whitening properties.

A Brief History of Oil Pulling and Coconut Oil

Oil pulling dates back about 2,500 years to Ayurveda which is traditional Indian medicine, that uses oil to nourish body tissues. Coconut oil, with its antimicrobial properties, is a staple in this practice. Studies show that oil pulling can have antimicrobial and antiinflammatory effects.

What is Oil Pulling?

Oil pulling is a method of cleansing the mouth using lipids, like coconut or sesame oil, to reduce bacteria. The single-cell structure of most oral bacteria allows fats to adhere to them, making it easier to flush them out. Coconut oil is particularly effective due to its lauric acid content, a natural antimicrobial agent that can help slow tooth decay. Typically, practitioners swish coconut oil for 20 minutes, but even 5 minutes can be beneficial. The recommended amount is between a teaspoon and a tablespoon.

Benefits of Coconut Oil for Teeth Whitening

- Soothes dry throats
- Heals dry, chapped lips
- Eliminates bad breath
- Easy to use and non-foaming
- Free from harmful chemicals
- Anti-inflammatory properties
- Promotes healing of bleeding gums

How to Use Coconut Oil to Whiten Teeth

1. **Take a Teaspoon of Coconut Oil:** Measure out a teaspoon. You should be using pure, organic, virgin, cold-pressed coconut oil.

2. **Liquefy the Oil in Your Mouth:** It will soften within seconds. Place the oil in your mouth and allow it to melt.
3. **Swish the Oil:** Swish for 5 minutes to start and work up to 20 minutes. Ensure it reaches all areas of your mouth. Avoid gargling. Do not swallow.
4. **Spit Out the Oil:** Spit into the trash to avoid clogging your sink.
5. **Rinse Your Mouth:** Rinse with still water to remove oily residue.
6. **Alternative Method:** Apply coconut oil to your toothbrush and brush your teeth as usual. In addition to Coconut Oil, you can also use Sunflower Oil or Sesame Oil.
7. **Scrape Your Tongue:** After oil pulling, use your tongue scraper as usual.

Side Effects
Some side effects include nausea, upset stomach, or an unpleasant taste, especially if the oil isn't properly spit out. Jaw fatigue or soreness can also occur from prolonged swishing. Occasionally, oil pulling can also trigger your gag reflex. If this happens, try leaning your head slightly forward and using less oil. Warming the oil can also make the oil thinner and less likely to cause you to gag.

On the Other Hand...
The devil's advocate says, there is another opinion on oil pulling. The "other side" says there are no reliable scientific studies to show that oil pulling reduces cavities, whitens teeth, or improves oral health and well-being. Based on the lack of scientific evidence, the American Dental Association does not recommend oil pulling as a dental hygiene practice.

Chief Smile Officer (you) 😊
Like anything that involves your health, you have to decide what is best for you. In today's healthcare environment, you have to look out for yourself. You are the Chief Advocate and Chief Smile Officer of yourself. You must always be advocating for yourself. Consult with your healthcare provider and dentist. Get on Google and do your own research. Ask your friends and family.

Olives

A Savory Secret for a Brighter Smile

Olives are not only a tasty snack but also a natural ally in your quest for whiter teeth. Rich in healthy fats and antioxidants, olives help promote overall oral health by supporting strong enamel and reducing plaque buildup. Their natural oils can assist in breaking down surface stains while their high fiber content stimulates saliva production, which helps cleanse your teeth and wash away food particles. Enjoy olives as part of your diet to enhance your oral care routine and achieve a naturally brighter, healthier smile!

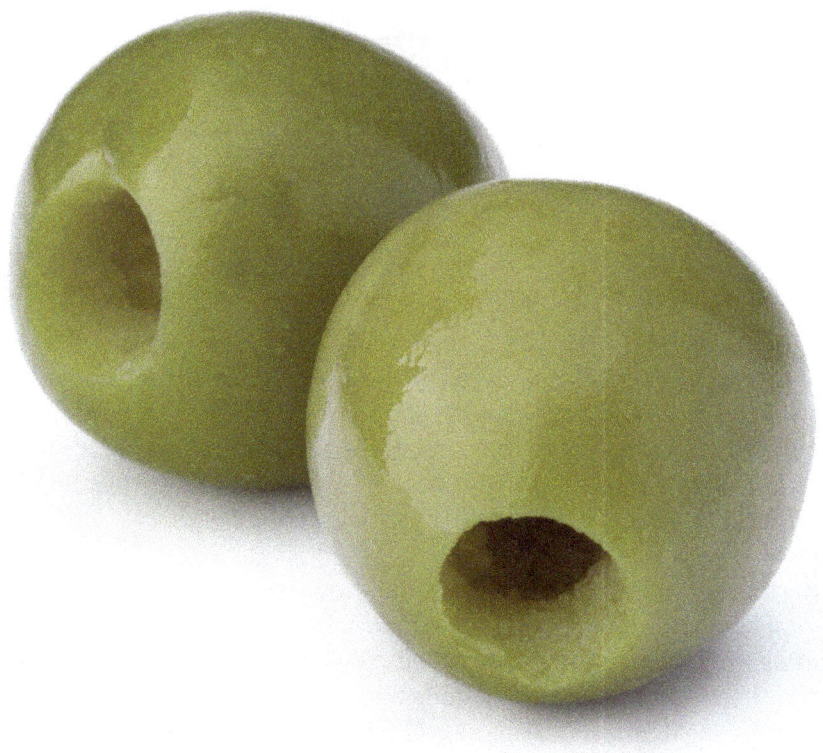

Onions

Bringing Tears of Joy to Your Smile!

Peeling Back the Layers:
Unveiling the Smile- Boosting Powers of Onions!

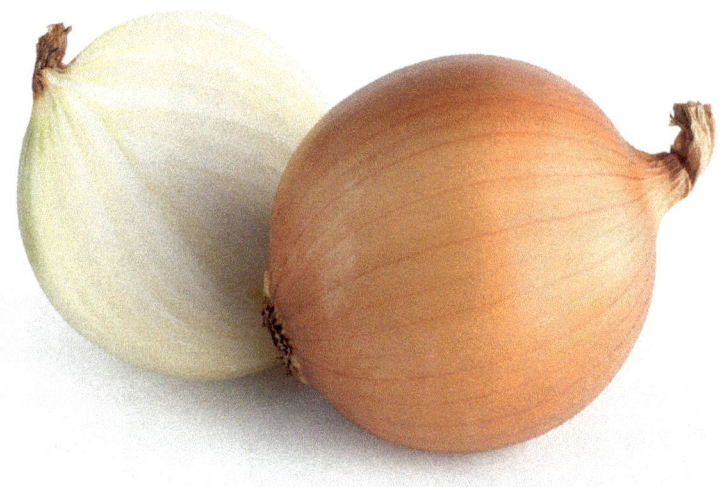

While onions are often associated with "onion breath," they possess remarkable benefits for oral health and bone strength. These humble vegetables contain sulfur, a crucial element necessary for the formation of connective tissue. Moreover, sulfur exhibits antibacterial properties, effectively inhibiting the formation of plaque.

Furthermore, onions contain a peptide known as GPCS, which plays a pivotal role in reducing bone breakdown. Embrace the multifaceted advantages of onions, not only for their culinary versatility but also for their contribution to a healthier smile and stronger bones.

Open Wide and Say 'Whiter Teeth!'

A beautiful smile begins with a healthy smile. Visit your dentist for regular checkups and professional cleanings. Dentists use abrasion and polishing techniques to effectively remove many stains caused by food and tobacco, helping you maintain a brighter smile.

As gone over here, a sensible, well-balanced diet can greatly impact your oral well-being. Eating healthy should be seen as an essential part of maintaining a beautiful smile, right alongside brushing and flossing."

Which leads me to remind you:
Don't Forget Daily Oral Care Maintenance

Maintaining white teeth can be as simple as daily brushing. Brush at least twice a day and floss once daily. For even better results, brush after every meal and snack. Regular brushing helps prevent stains and yellowing, especially along the gum line. Electric and sonic toothbrushes may be more effective than traditional ones in removing plaque and surface stains.

> *A Beautiful Smile Begins With a Healthy Smile*

Orange

Don't Throw the Peel Away

A 2010 study reported that eating fruit daily is the best way to whiten teeth using your diet. Researchers tried various methods for three months and determined that strawberries, orange peels, and lemon juice were some of the most effective whiteners you could use. All have enzymes and acids that help break down stains. Just be careful, as too much acid can wear away enamel, so always follow with a glass of water.

Orange You Glad?
Exploring the Zesty Benefits of a Brighter Smile!

Discover the natural secret to brighter, whiter teeth with the power of orange peels. Renowned for their safe and effective whitening properties, the inside of an orange peel contains limonene, a natural solvent cleaner also found in many commercial teeth whitening products.

Unlike the acidic flesh of the fruit, the white part of the peel, known as the albedo, poses no risk to tooth enamel, ensuring a gentle yet powerful whitening experience. Even dentists recommend utilizing the toothfriendly benefits of orange peels, advising against common foods that can harm your teeth.

Unlock the full potential of orange peel whitening by incorporating both the peel and its stringy white portion into your dental routine. Simply rub the inside of the peel directly onto your teeth to witness their natural brilliance. For added effectiveness, blend the orange peel with crushed bay leaves and apply the mixture for enhanced whitening results.

Embrace the holistic approach to oral care by utilizing every part of the orange, including its peel. Contrary to popular belief, orange peels are not acidic like other citrus fruits, offering a rich source of vitamin C as a gentle alternative to harsh chemical whiteners. Safeguard your enamel by incorporating this natural remedy into your daily regimen, combating tartar buildup and minimizing plaque for a radiant smile.

Packed with vitamin C and bursting with flavor, oranges serve as more than just a nutritious snack—they double as a potent teeth whitener. Research indicates that the enzyme bromelain found in oranges acts as a natural stain remover, effectively breaking down plaque and preventing dental decay.

Elevate your dental care routine with the power of oranges, unlocking a brighter, healthier smile the natural way.

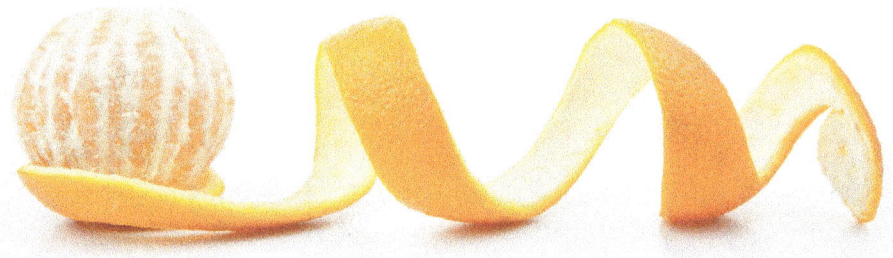

P

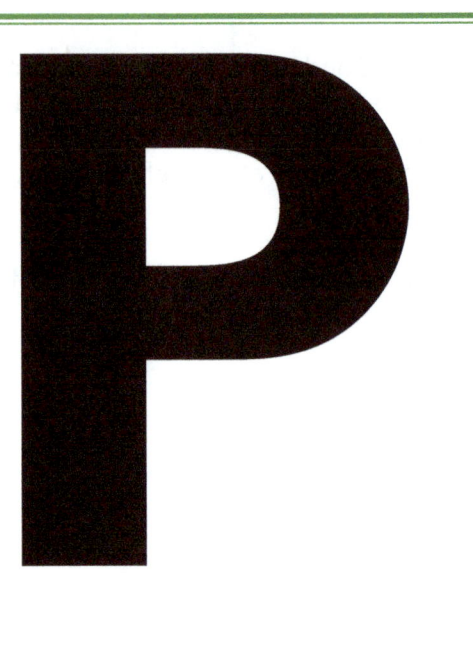

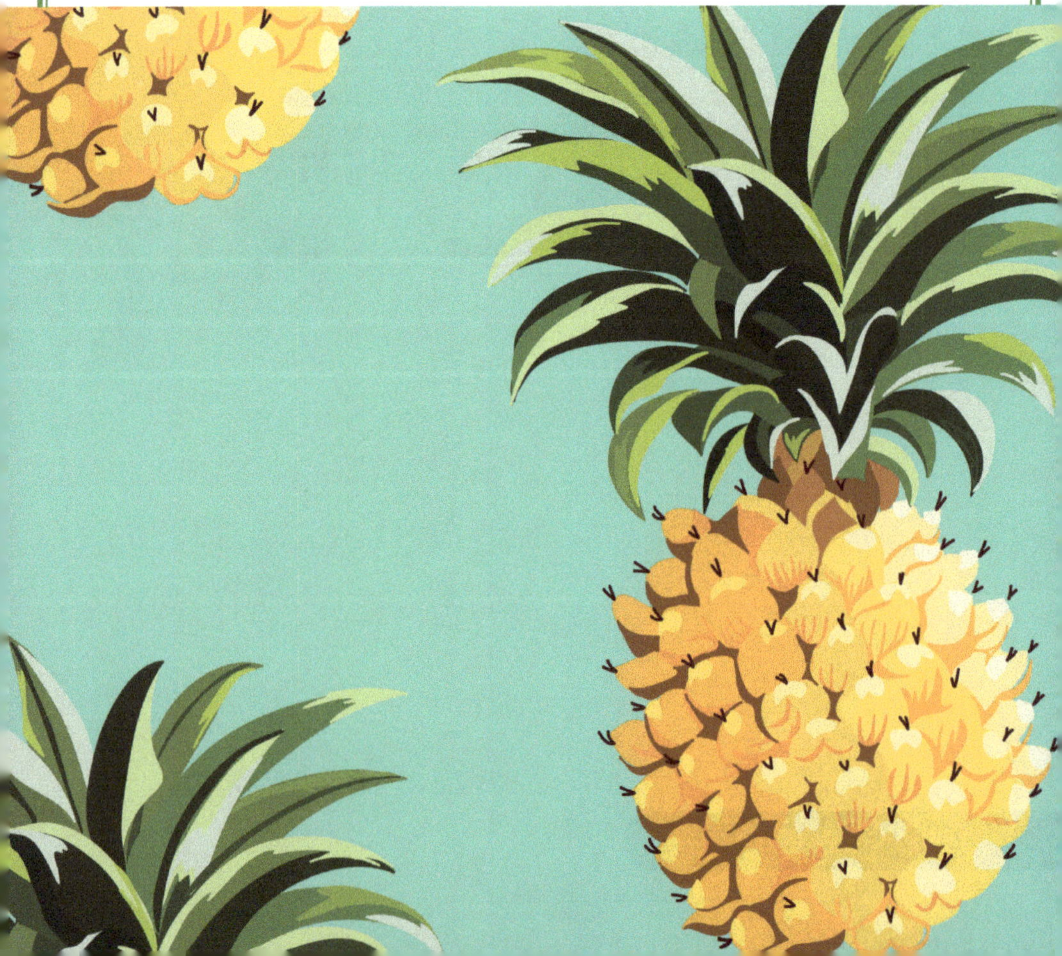

Papayas

A Tropical Delight for a Brighter Smile

Papayas are more than just a delicious tropical fruit—they also aid in naturally whitening your teeth. Rich in the enzyme papain, papayas help break down proteins and remove surface stains, promoting a cleaner, brighter smile. Their high vitamin C content supports gum health and strengthens enamel, while their natural sweetness provides a refreshing treat without contributing to tooth discoloration. Enjoy papayas as a nutritious snack or in your favorite dishes to enhance your oral care routine and maintain a naturally radiant smile!

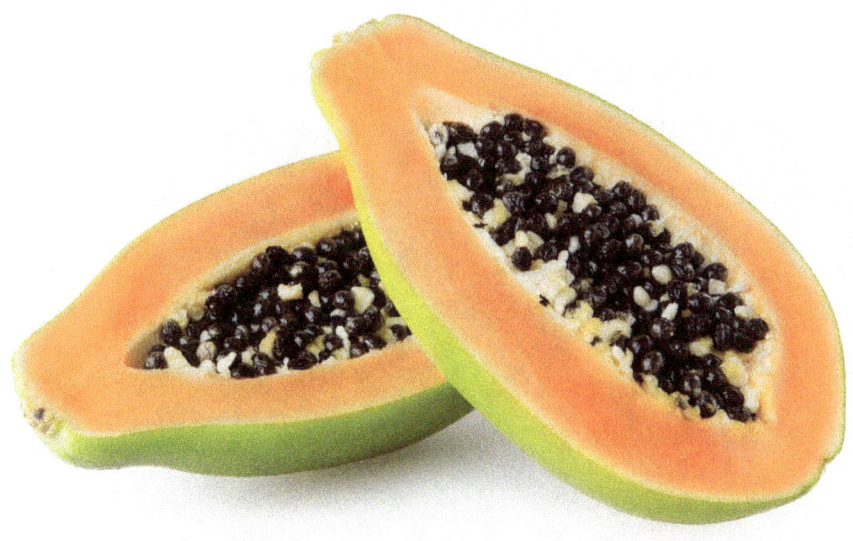

Parsley

A Fresh Herb for a Brighter Smile

Parsley is not just a garnish—it's a natural helper for whitening your teeth. This vibrant herb contains compounds that neutralize bad breath and its natural chlorophyll acts as a gentle cleanser, helping to remove surface stains. Parsley also promotes saliva production, which assists in washing away food particles and bacteria that can lead to discoloration. Add parsley to your meals or chew on fresh leaves to enjoy its refreshing benefits and support a naturally brighter, healthier smile!

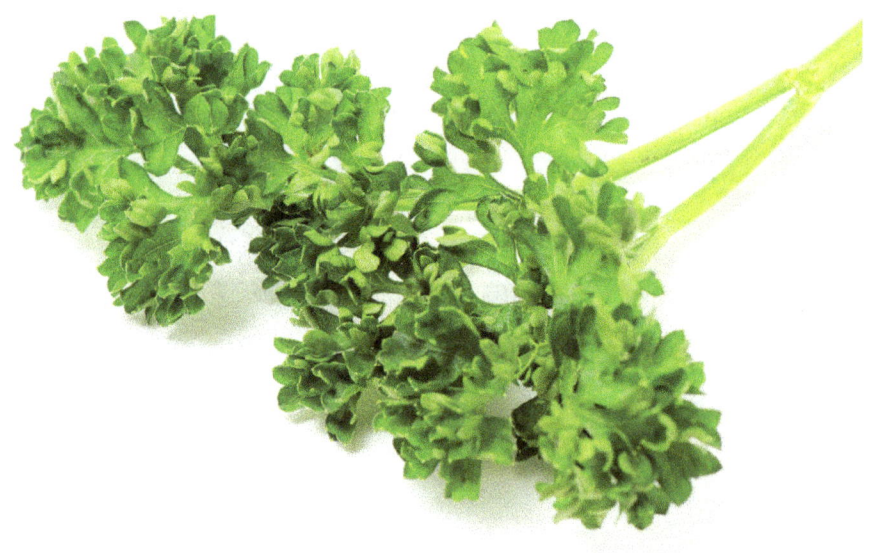

Peas

A Tiny Green Powerhouse for a Brighter Smile

Peas might be small, but they pack a big punch when it comes to natural teeth whitening. Rich in vitamins and minerals, peas support strong enamel and overall oral health. Their high fiber content stimulates saliva production, which helps cleanse your teeth by washing away food particles and reducing plaque buildup.

Additionally, the natural crunchiness of peas provides a gentle scrubbing effect, helping to remove surface stains. Incorporate these little green gems into your diet for a nutritious boost and a naturally whiter, healthier smile!

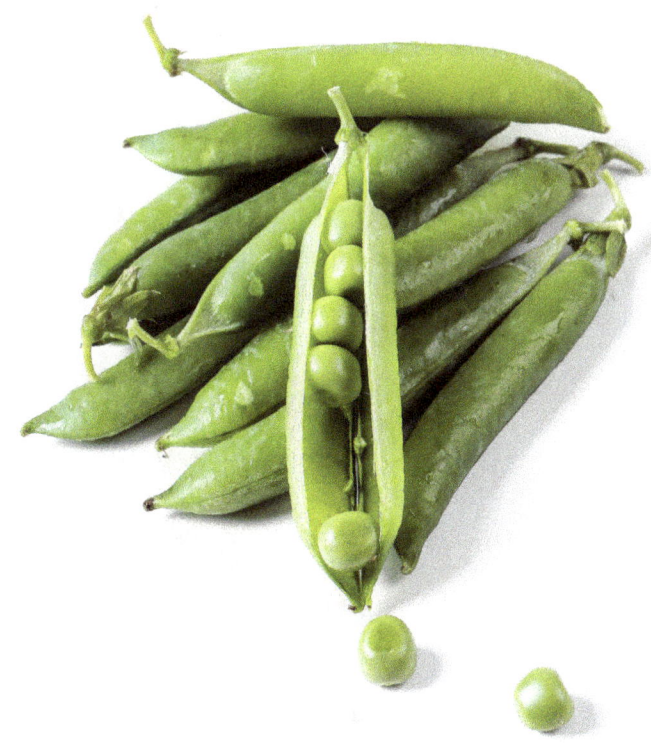

Peaches

A Juicy Treat for a Brighter Smile

Peaches are not only a delicious fruit but also a natural ally for whitening your teeth. Their high water content helps stimulate saliva production, which aids in washing away food particles and reducing plaque buildup. Rich in vitamins and antioxidants, peaches support gum health and strengthen enamel, contributing to a naturally brighter smile. Enjoy fresh peaches as a sweet, nutritious snack or add them to your meals to enhance your oral care routine and keep your smile shining!

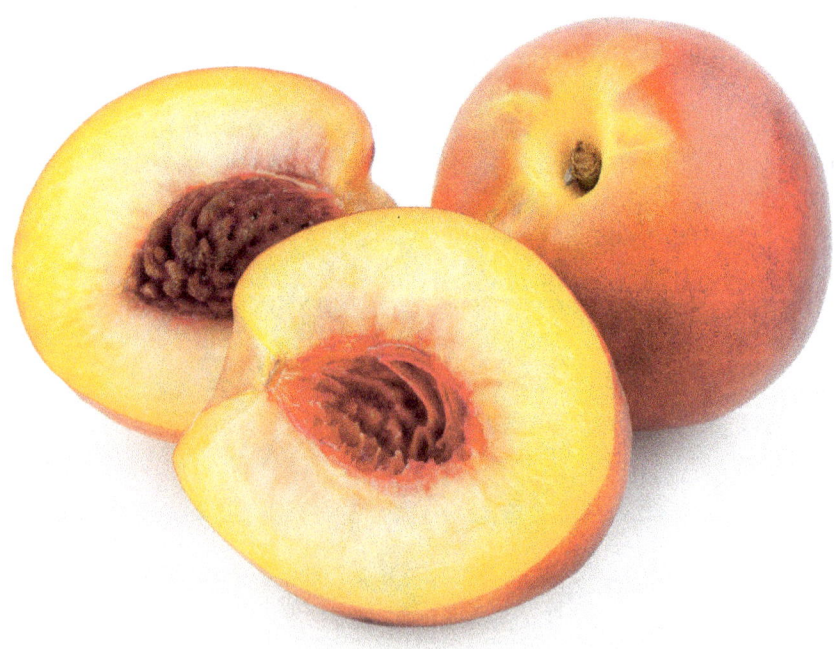

Pears

Pear-ly Whites: Discovering the Juicy Secrets of Pears for a Radiant Smile

Discover the refreshing benefits of pears for promoting oral health and teeth whitening. Pears are renowned for their juicy and flavorful nature, stimulating saliva production. Enjoying pears can also help neutralize bacteria in the mouth that may contribute to staining, supporting efforts to maintain a bright, white smile.

Classified as a Foundation Food, pears offer essential nutrients for overall health. Rich in polyphenols, they provide antioxidant support, protecting the teeth and gums from damage caused by free radicals. Pears also contain boron, a trace mineral vital for bone metabolism. Working alongside Vitamin D, boron helps reduce urinary excretion of calcium and magnesium, supporting optimal bone health and strength. Incorporate pears into your diet to nourish your smile from within, embracing their alkalizing properties and nutrient-rich profile.

In the realm of smile-inducing foods, few have earned the title of "gift of the gods" quite like the pear. Revered by the ancient Greeks and Romans, this versatile fruit has been celebrated throughout history, from classic works of art to beloved holiday tunes like "The Twelve Days of Christmas."

Explore the whitening benefits of crunchy pears. Their fibrous texture can scrub away surface stains while their natural sweetness satisfies cravings for sugary treats.

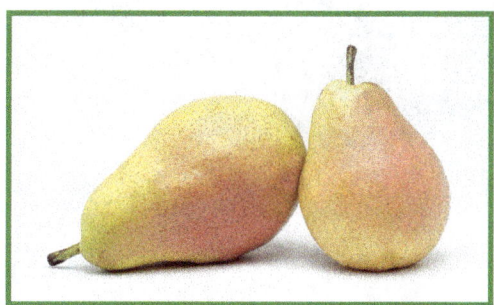

Peppers

Snack on crisp, raw bell peppers to boost saliva production and promote cleaner, whiter teeth. Their high water content also helps rinse away food particles and stains.

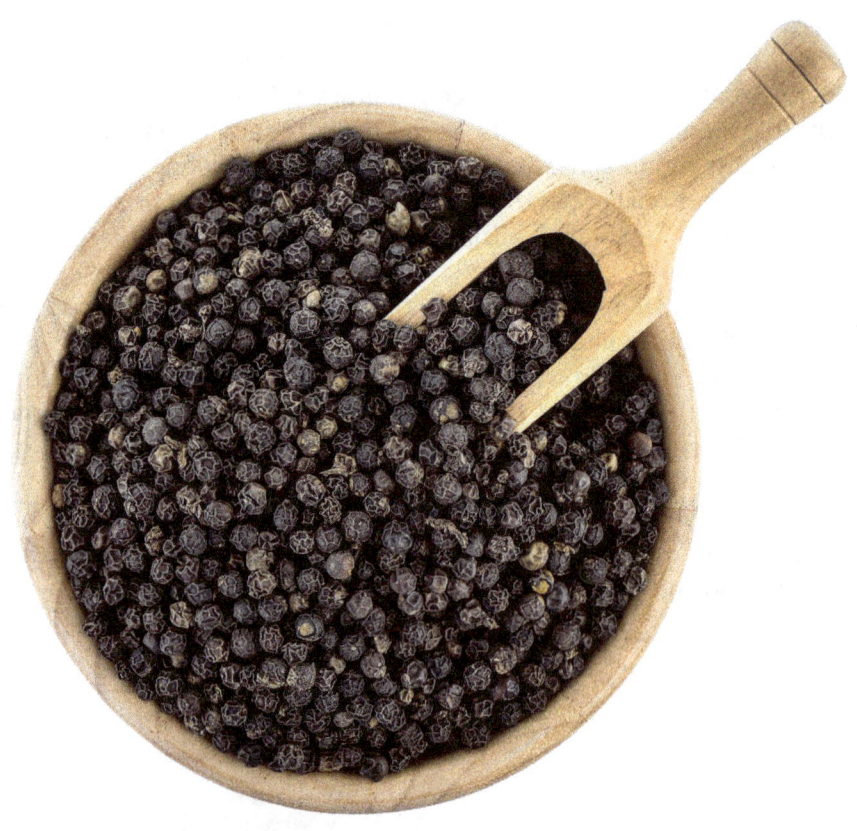

Pineapple

Tropical Smile - Unveiling the Sweet Secrets of Pineapple for a Brighter Grin!

Include pineapple in your diet for its enzyme bromelain, which can help break down stains and promote a brighter smile.

Unlock the natural stain-fighting power of pineapple, a remarkable fruit renowned for its ability to remove dental discoloration. What sets pineapple apart is its rich content of "bromelain," a potent mixture of natural enzymes primarily known for digesting proteins, yet also offering numerous health benefits. In a noteworthy 2011 study, toothpaste containing bromelain extract demonstrated significant stain removal efficacy compared to a control substance, showcasing the remarkable potential of this enzyme in enhancing dental aesthetics. Embrace the whitening prowess of pineapple and harness the benefits of bromelain for a brighter, more radiant smile.

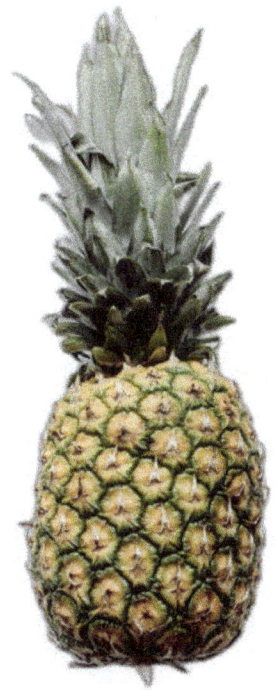

The Power of Smiling

Your Key to Happiness and Well-Being

In a world where happiness can sometimes feel as elusive as a pot of gold at the end of a rainbow, neuroscience offers a surprising revelation: the simple act of smiling can be as uplifting as indulging in 2,000 chocolate bars or receiving a windfall of $25,000 cash. Yes, you read that right.

Expert Melanie Curtin sheds light on a groundbreaking study conducted in the UK, where researchers utilized cutting-edge technology to gauge the impact of various stimuli on participants' moods. What emerged as the ultimate mood enhancer? None other than the humble smile.

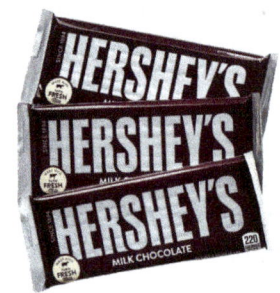

Digging deeper into the science behind this phenomenon, it's revealed that smiling triggers remarkable effects within the brain. Regardless of your current emotional state, flashing a grin prompts the brain to release feel-good hormones, effectively boosting your mood. So, even on those gloomy days, a smile has the power to lift your spirits, validating the age-old advice to "fake it til you make it." But the benefits of smiling extend far beyond momentary happiness. Studies have linked smiling to longevity, with beaming individuals outliving their unsmiling counterparts by a significant margin.

Moreover, the width of one's smile serves as a telling indicator of future success, influencing everything from personal relationships to professional endeavors.

Interestingly, the perception of a smile goes a long way in shaping interpersonal interactions. Not only are smiling individuals viewed as more likable and approachable but they're also deemed more competent—a valuable asset in any social or professional setting. Curious about your smiling habits? Statistics reveal intriguing insights, with children leading the pack with an impressive 400 smiles per day. While over 30% of adults smile more than 20 times daily, those who grin less than five times a day may want to reconsider their approach to happiness.

In essence, the science is clear: smiling isn't just a fleeting expression; it's a gateway to enhanced well-being and a brighter outlook on life. So, the next time you're feeling down, remember the transformative power of a smile—it may just be the key to unlocking your happiness potential.

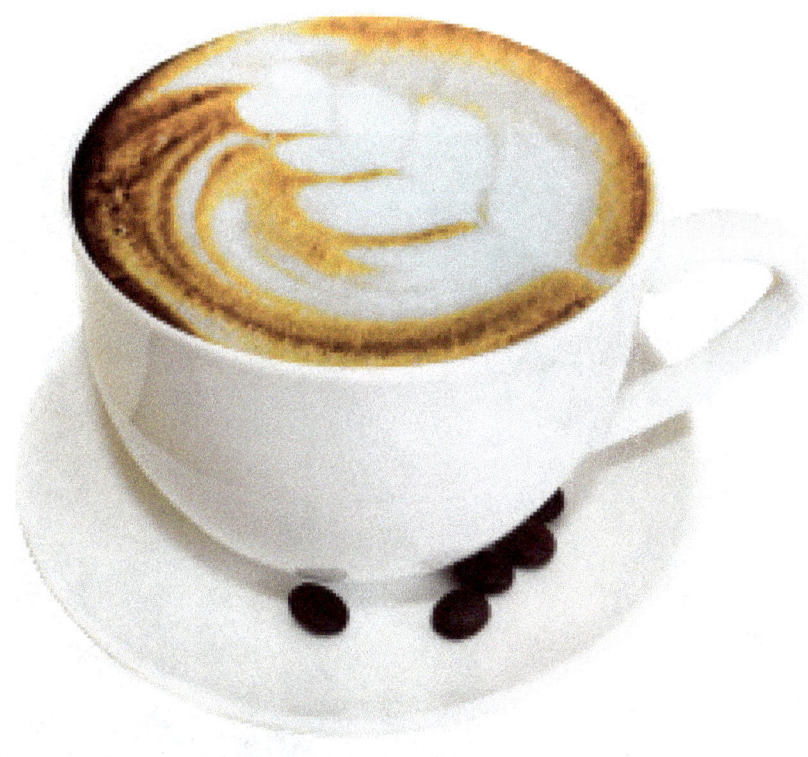

R

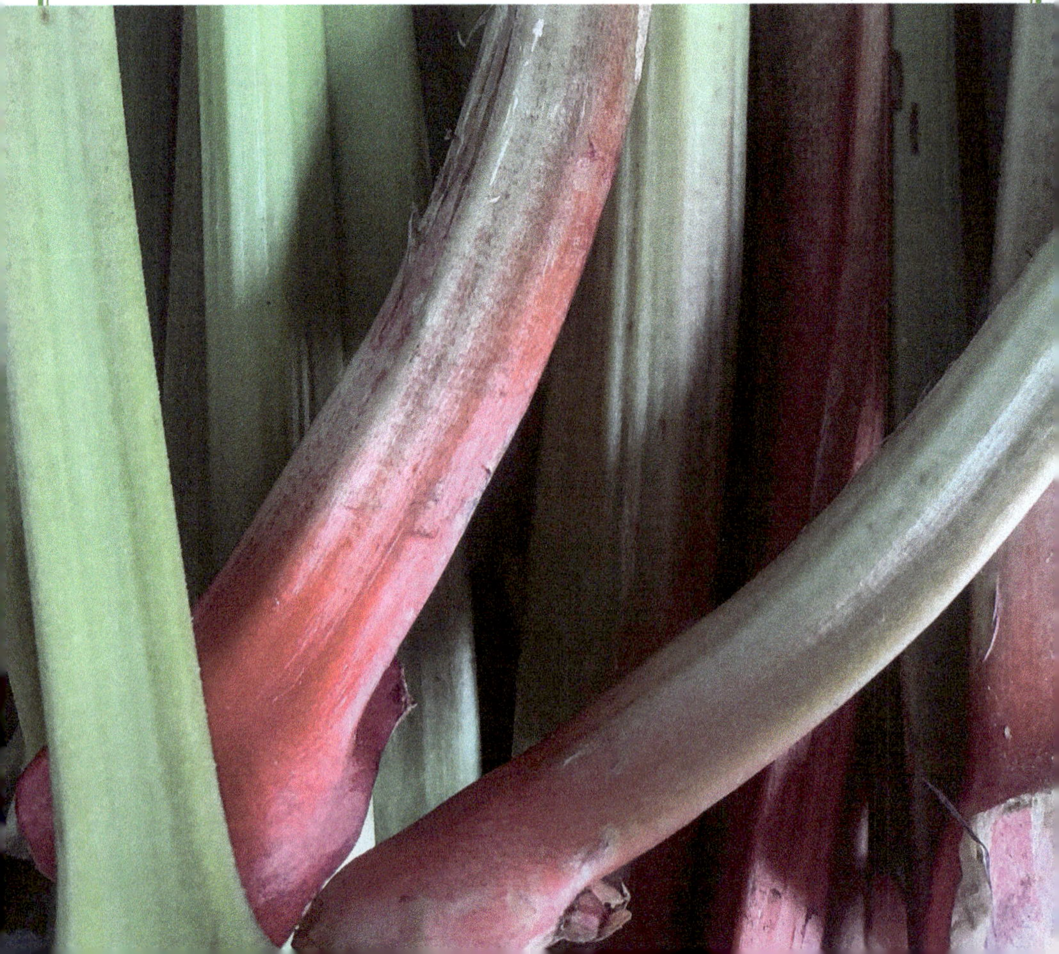

Radishes

A Crisp Secret for a Brighter Smile

Radishes are more than just a crunchy addition to your salads— they also support natural teeth whitening. Their crisp texture acts as a natural scrubber, helping to dislodge food particles and reduce plaque buildup. Radishes are rich in vitamin C and antioxidants, which support gum health and strengthen enamel. Additionally, their high water content stimulates saliva production, aiding in the natural cleansing of your teeth. Enjoy radishes as a fresh snack or in your meals to enhance your oral care routine and achieve a naturally brighter, healthier smile!

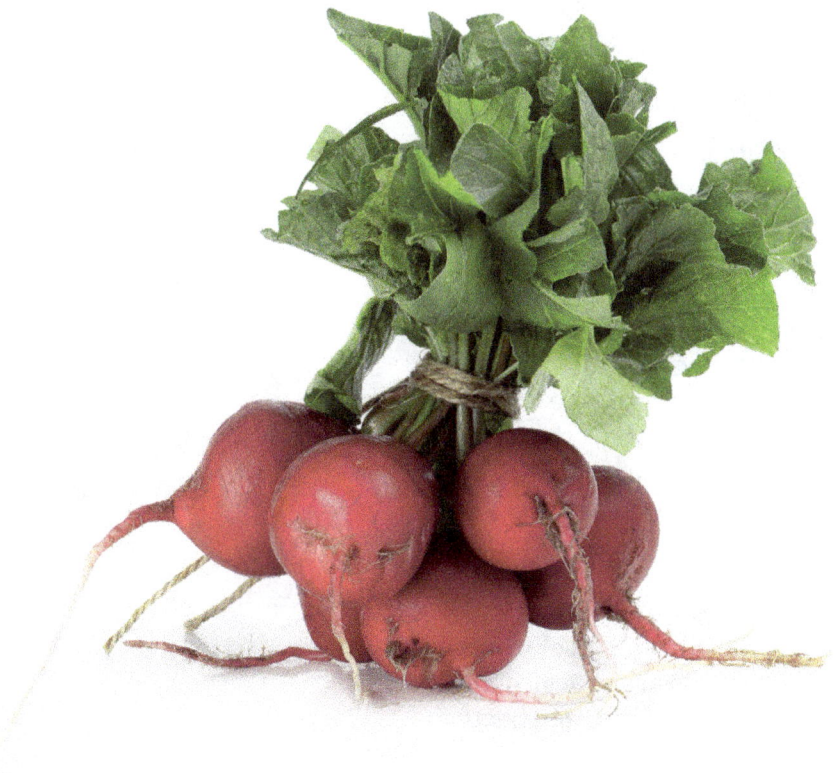

Raisins

Raisin' the Bar - Unveiling the Sweet Secrets of Raisins for a Brighter Smile!

Contrary to what one might expect, sticky and sweet raisins can actually benefit your oral health.

Researchers at the University of Illinois at Chicago's College of Dentistry have discovered that raisins may improve oral health outcomes.

In a study presented at the annual meeting of the American Society for Microbiology, it was found that oleanolic acid, a compound present in seedless raisins, has the potential to inhibit the growth of two types of harmful oral bacteria: Streptococcus mutans, known for causing cavities, and Porphyromonas gingivalis, associated with periodontal disease.

Beyond its cavity-fighting properties, oleanolic acid also aids in protecting teeth from the accumulation of plaque. Embrace the surprising benefits of raisins as a natural ally in maintaining a healthy and bright smile.

You may think raisins are bad for your teeth because of their sticky sweetness, but they're actually protective. Research shows that bran cereal with raisins helps clean the mouth faster than the same cereal without raisins. Chewing raisins stimulates saliva, which helps prevent plaque, stains, and cavities from developing by neutralizing the acidic environment created by other foods and bacteria in your mouth.

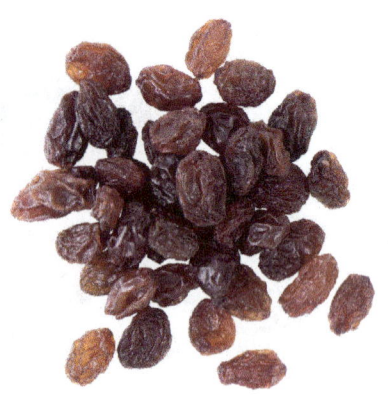

Raspberries

A Berry Delight for a Brighter Smile

Raspberries are not only a tasty fruit but also a natural ally in your quest for whiter teeth. Rich in antioxidants and vitamin C, raspberries help support gum health and strengthen enamel. Their natural acidity and high fiber content work together to gently break down surface stains and promote saliva production, which aids in washing away food particles and reducing plaque buildup. Enjoy raspberries as a sweet and refreshing snack or in your favorite dishes to enhance your oral care routine and achieve a naturally brighter, healthier smile!

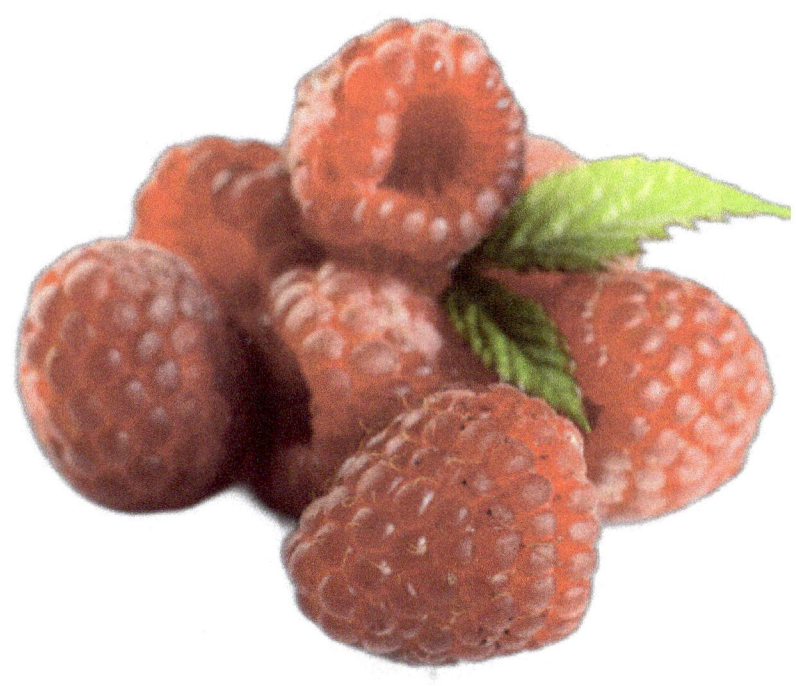

Rhubarb

Nature's Smile Brightener

Rhubarb is often celebrated for its tart taste and versatility in the kitchen, but did you know it's also a surprising ally in the quest for a brighter smile? Let's dive into the reasons why rhubarb is a fantastic addition to your oral hygiene routine.

A Natural Cleanser

Rhubarb is packed with natural acids that act as gentle cleansers for your teeth. The oxalic acid found in rhubarb can help break down and remove stains on your teeth, giving them a whiter appearance. While too much acid can be harmful, the moderate amounts in rhubarb are just right for promoting a cleaner, brighter smile when consumed in balance with other foods.

Rich in Vitamin C

This vibrant plant is an excellent source of vitamin C, an essential nutrient that plays a significant role in oral health. Vitamin C helps strengthen your gums and teeth by promoting collagen production, which is crucial for maintaining healthy gum tissue. A strong foundation is key to showcasing those pearly whites!

Encourages Saliva Production

Eating rhubarb can stimulate saliva production, which is a natural defense against plaque buildup and cavities. Saliva helps wash away food particles and neutralizes acids in the mouth, reducing the risk of tooth decay. A well-moistened mouth not only feels fresher but also keeps your smile brighter.

Antioxidant Powerhouse

Rhubarb is also rich in antioxidants, which help combat free radicals in the body. These free radicals can contribute to gum disease and other oral health issues. By including rhubarb in your diet, you are helping protect your gums and teeth from harmful oxidative stress.

How to Enjoy Rhubarb for Your Smile
- **Rhubarb Smoothies:** Blend rhubarb with your favorite fruits and a touch of honey for a refreshing, smile-friendly drink.
- **Rhubarb Compote:** Use as a topping for yogurt or oatmeal to add a tangy twist to your breakfast.
- **Rhubarb Tea:** Brew rhubarb stalks for a tart tea that promotes hydration and oral health.

A Note of Caution
While rhubarb offers many benefits for oral health, it's important to remember that moderation is key. Rhubarb leaves contain high levels of oxalic acid and should not be consumed. Stick to the stalks and enjoy them as part of a balanced diet to reap the dental benefits without any drawbacks.

Conclusion
Rhubarb may not be the first food that comes to mind when thinking about oral hygiene, but its natural cleansing properties, vitamin C content, and ability to boost saliva production make it a great addition to your diet for a brighter smile. So next time you're looking for a unique way to care for your teeth, consider reaching for some rhubarb and enjoy its delightful benefits.

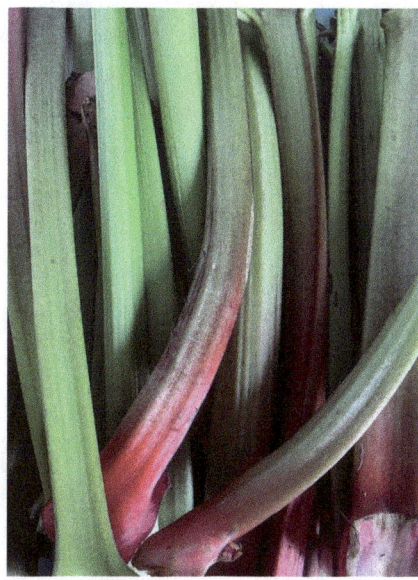

S

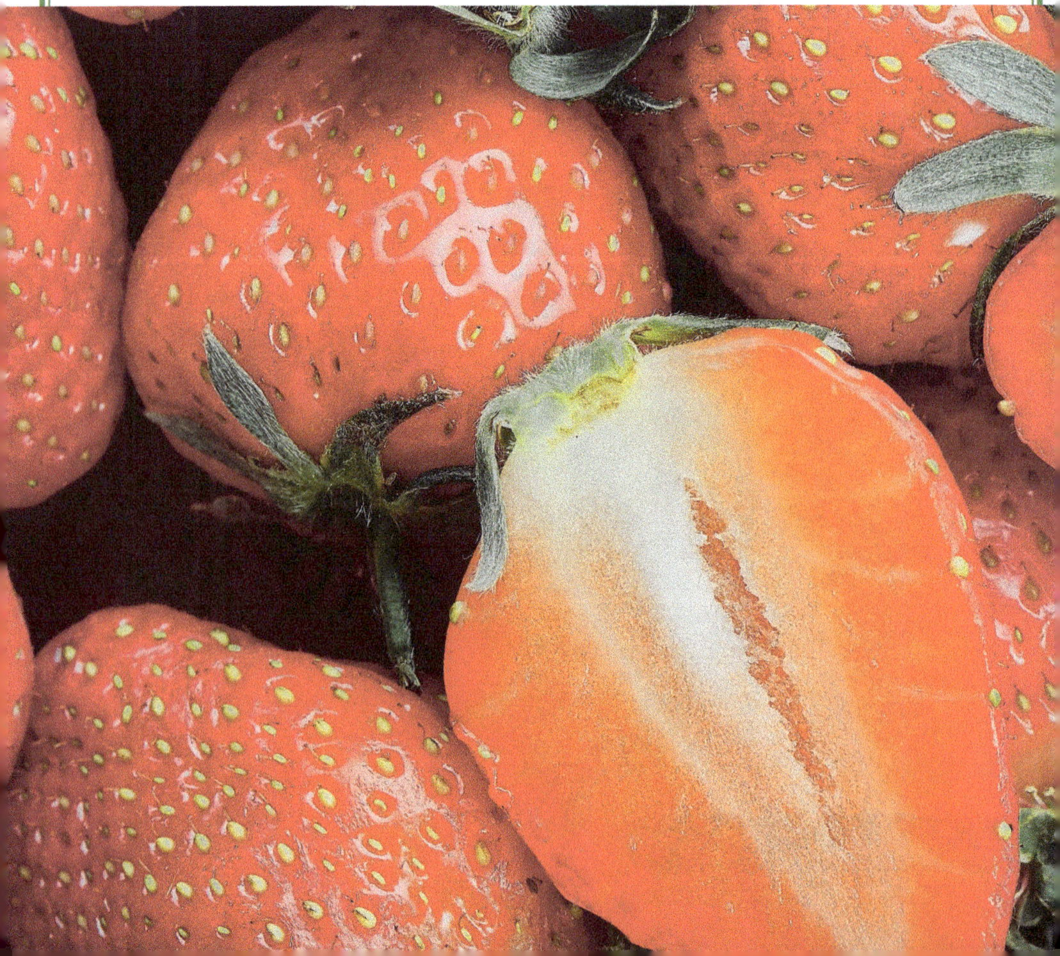

Sage

A Natural Ally for a Brighter Smile

Sage is a versatile herb renowned for its healing properties. Rich in natural oils and compounds, sage can help remove stains from teeth, making it a powerful ally in your quest for a whiter smile.

According to a study in the Journal of Traditional and Complementary Medicine, sage's antibacterial properties also play a significant role in maintaining oral hygiene and potentially whitening teeth.

How to Use Sage for Teeth Whitening

1. **Fresh Sage Leaves:** Crush fresh sage leaves and rub them directly onto your teeth.
2. **Sage Powder:** Dry sage leaves, grind them into a powder, and use it as a toothpaste.

Regular use of sage can contribute to a cleaner, whiter smile. Embrace the natural benefits of this amazing herb for a healthier, brighter you.

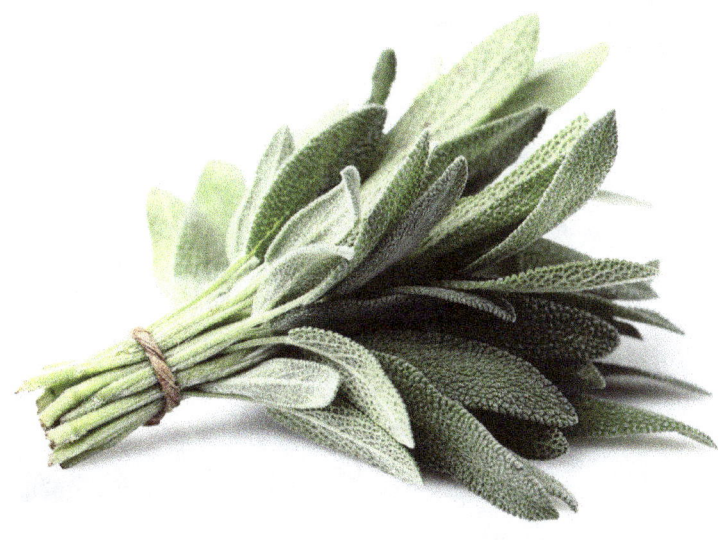

Sauces

Beware!

Soy sauce and tomato sauce, as well as other deeply colored sauces, are believed to have significant staining potential.

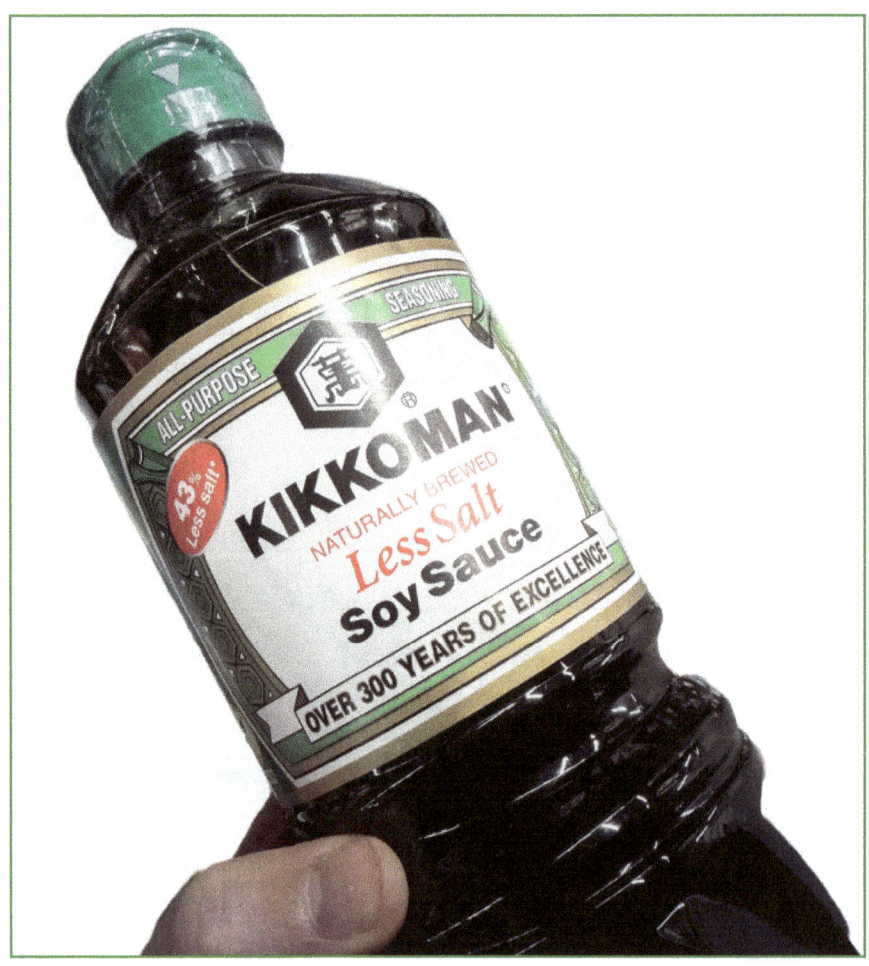

Seeds

Chia, Chia, Chia!

Incorporate crunchy seeds like flaxseeds and chia seeds into your meals for a teeth-friendly source of omega-3 fatty acids. Their abrasive texture can help remove plaque and surface stains.

Incorporating these seeds into your diet can help remove surface stains and reveal a whiter smile. Sesame seeds serve as an excellent gentle exfoliant for your teeth.

The gritty texture of sunflower seeds serves as a natural exfoliator for your teeth, helping to remove surface stains and leave your smile looking brighter. Similarly, almonds, walnuts, and cashews offer an abrasive quality that aids in the removal of plaque and other stain-causing substances, promoting a cleaner and healthier oral environment.

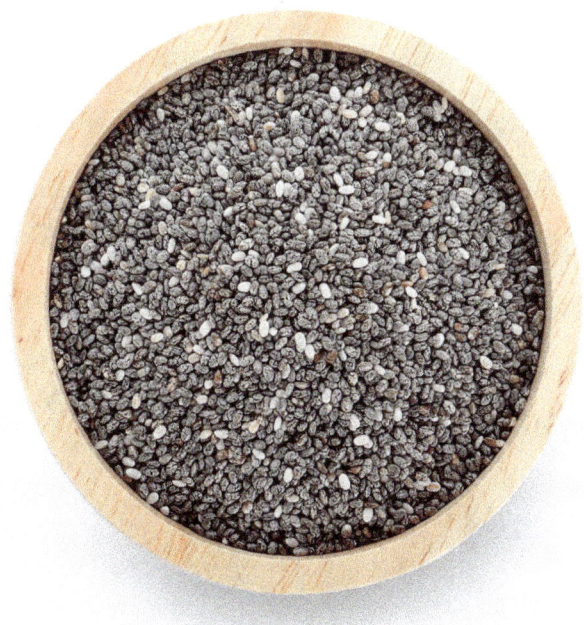

Shiitake Mushrooms

A Savory Boost for a Brighter Smile

Shiitake mushrooms are more than just a flavorful addition to your dishes—they also contribute to natural teeth whitening. Rich in lentinans and other compounds, shiitake mushrooms help reduce plaque and prevent the buildup of harmful bacteria in the mouth.

Their natural properties can assist in maintaining strong enamel and promoting overall oral health. Including shiitake mushrooms in your diet supports a cleaner mouth and contributes to a naturally brighter, healthier smile, making them a delicious and beneficial choice for your oral care routine.

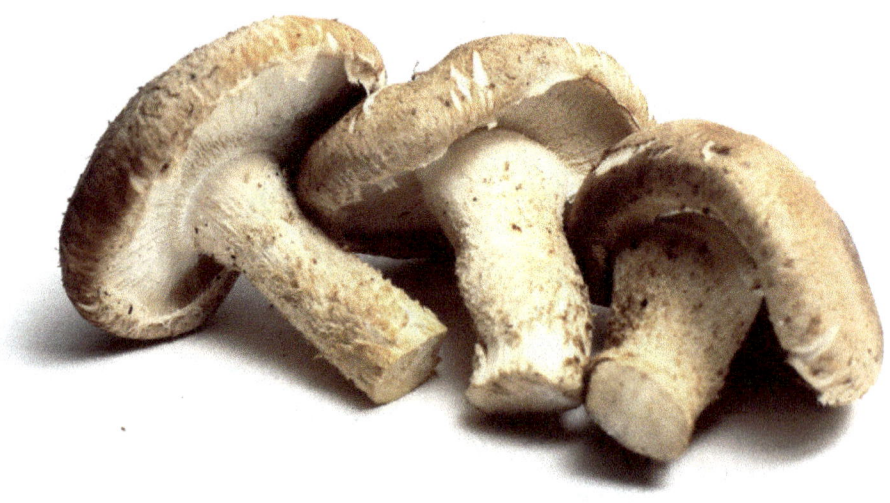

Smoking

To Keep Teeth White - Don't Light

Smoking not only harms your health but also stands out as a leading cause of teeth staining. In fact, I'd argue there's nothing worse. It's the smile's nemesis. Fortunately, high-quality teeth whitening can reverse the cosmetic effects of smoking. Tobacco stains, with their brown hue, penetrate enamel's tiny crevices, proving resistant to scrubbing.

Whether it's cigarettes, cigars, vaping, or chewing tobacco, the nicotine and tar in these products create a yellow or brownish discoloration that's difficult to remove. This staining is more than just surface deep; it can penetrate the tiny pores in your enamel, leading to long-term and stubborn stains.

Over time, these stains become deeply embedded. Furthermore, smoking contributes to bad breath, and gum disease, and increases the risk of several cancers. Tobacco use also poses significant risks to your overall oral health, including gum disease and oral cancer, which further impact the appearance of your teeth.

I personally, strongly advocate for quitting the use of tobacco, not only for the sake of a brighter smile but also for your dental and overall health.

For those looking to reverse tobacco-related teeth staining, only use high-quality teeth whitening treatments, and a strict oral hygiene routine is often necessary to combat the effects of this smile nemesis.

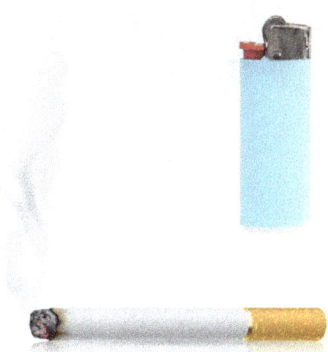

Spices

Spice Up Your Smile!

Uncover how spices like turmeric and cinnamon possess natural whitening properties, leaving your teeth sparkling and your taste buds tingling. These spices contain compounds like curcumin and cinnamic aldehyde, which not only lead you on a flavorful adventure but have also been linked to tooth whitening.

The Great Debate

Straw or No Straw? The Smile Saga Unveiled!
Enhance Your Smile with Straws!

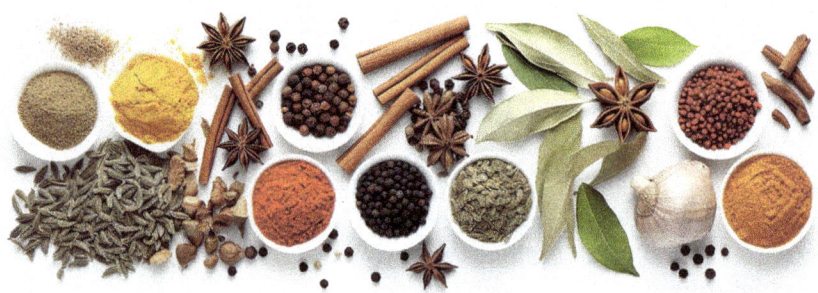

Sip and Smile

Unveiling the Sipping Secrets of Straws for a Whiter Grin!

Discover how sipping through a straw can be a game-changer for your dental health—it's like a tiny superhero for your teeth!

The Bright Side of Using Straws

Picture this: you enjoy your favorite acidic drink without worrying about the aftermath on your sparkling smile. Straws swoop in to save the day by diverting those potentially staining liquids away from your front teeth.

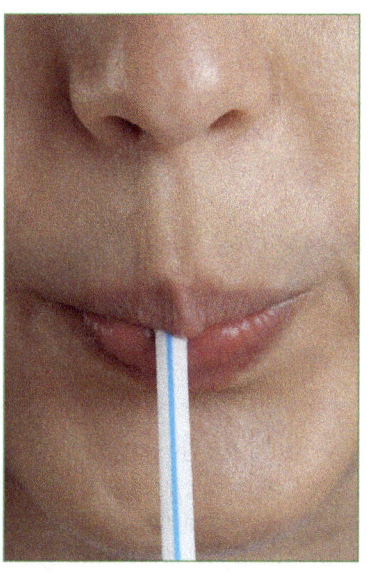

But wait, there's more! (Since the first time I heard Ron Popeil say that I've always wanted to say it too :) With a little strategic placement, straws can shield your back teeth from the perils of sugar and acid attacks. It's like creating a fortress of protection for your precious enamel!. But wait, there's more fun to be had! Sipping on water through a straw not only quenches your thirst but also gives your teeth a mini spa treatment, washing away pesky debris and bacteria like a refreshing wave of oral bliss.

The Flip Side of the Straw Story

Now, let's not get too carried away with our straw adventures. Mischievous straws, when not properly positioned, might accidentally cause trouble for your front teeth by creating little pools of sugary and acidic liquids. Talk about a dental conundrum!

And here's the scoop: relying solely on straws won't magically make sugary drinks tooth-friendly. It's like trying to hide from the dentist behind a flimsy straw curtain—it just doesn't work!

Oh, and one more thing—those sneaky sugary sips can still wreak havoc on your teeth, even if you're sipping through a straw. It's like a stealthy dental ninja attack that your teeth aren't prepared for!

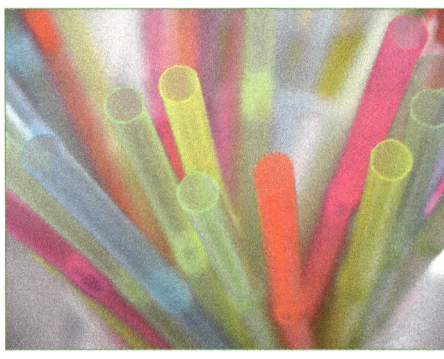

Choose Your Sips Wisely!
Whether you're sipping through a straw or going au naturel, be a smile superhero by picking smile-friendly beverages like water. And when you do indulge in the occasional treat, wield your straw like a dental knight, positioning it to minimize any potential tooth tussles. Your smile will thank you for it!

WhiteDiet: Now it is time to switch over to the WhiteDiet.

For at least the first 48 hours after whitening, you should choose foods and drinks that are white or pale. This will help to avoid any stains developing, while also preventing any further irritation to your teeth. and gums. Drinking plenty of water will help your gum tissue to recover quicker.

Seaweed

Sea-licious Smiles: Unveiling the Ocean's Secret Weapon for Whiter Teeth

Elevate your sushi night with an unexpected benefit: seaweed. In addition to its delicious taste, seaweed contains bacterial enzymes that actively combat plaque buildup, promoting a natural whitening effect on teeth. If sushi isn't your preference, fear not!

Baked seaweed snacks offer the same dental benefits while providing a healthier alternative to traditional potato chips.

Say goodbye to excess sodium and artificial ingredients, and indulge in the wholesome goodness of seaweed for a brighter smile and a guiltfree snack option.

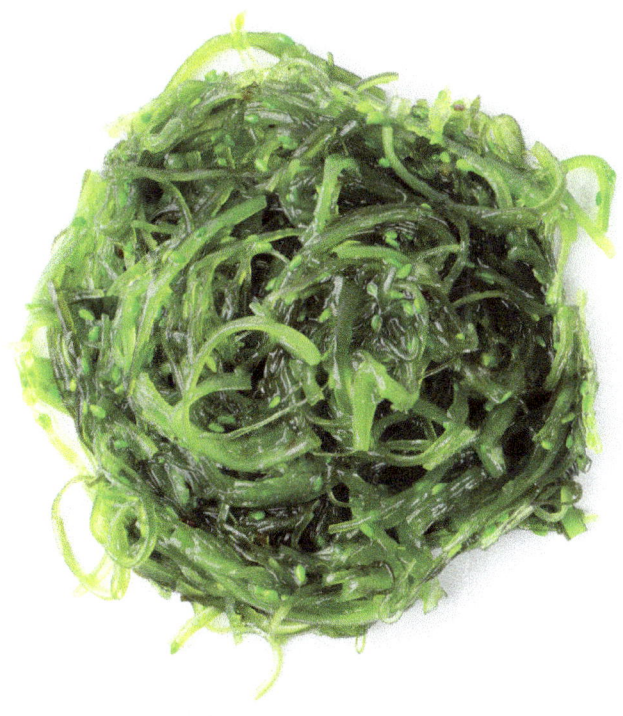

Sesame

Nature's Scrubbing Toothbrush

These will help in the reduction of plaque deposits. Just take a few teaspoons of sesame seeds a few times per week, and you will begin to note a change in how clean your teeth are. Your dentist will also probably see reduced plaque deposits.

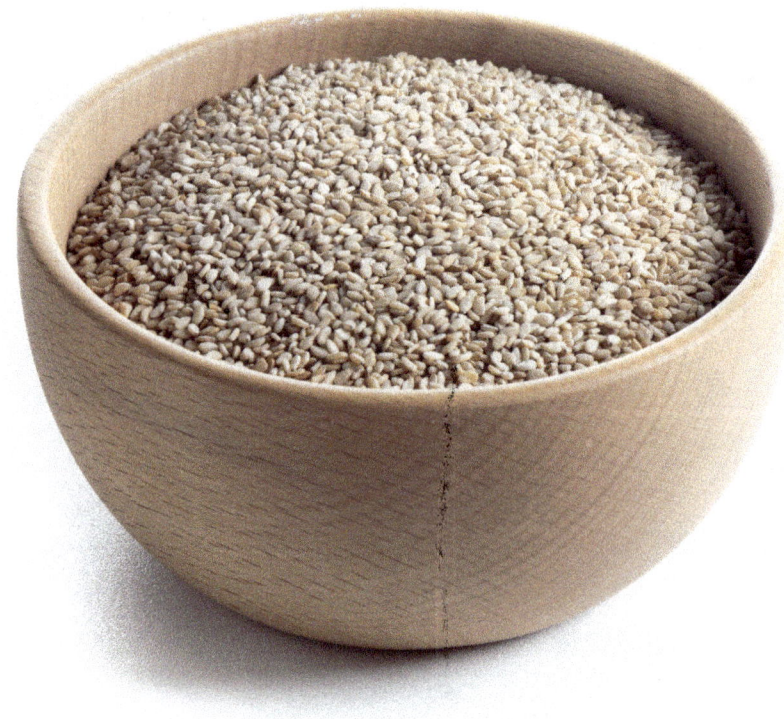

Strawberries

Berry Bright Smiles - Unveiling the Sweet Secrets of Strawberries

Unveil the hidden potential of strawberries for enhancing oral health and brightening your smile, Malic acid, a primary component of strawberries, acts as a natural astringent, effectively removing surface tooth discoloration.

Whether enjoyed in salads, desserts, or cereal, incorporating strawberries into your diet can lead to a brighter smile. You can even maximize their whitening effects by mashing them up and applying them directly to your toothbrush.

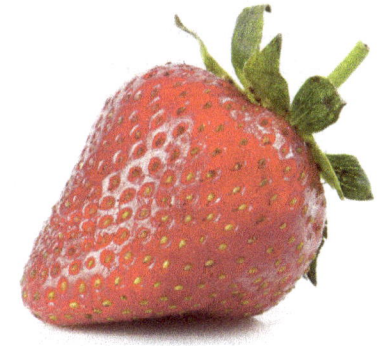

Beyond their delectable taste, strawberries contain malic acids, which play a crucial role in converting carbohydrates into energy for muscles. Maintaining adequate levels of malic acids is vital for robust dental health, as these acids can dissolve superficial stains on the teeth's surface.

If strawberries aren't your preference, fret not! Malic acid can also be found in apples, nectarines, cherries, bananas, peaches, and lychee. So, indulge in these fruits to reap the oral health benefits and achieve a whiter, brighter, healthier smile.

Blueberries, raspberries, cranberries, cherries, and their berry brethren are undeniably beneficial for your overall health packing a lot of nutrients in a small package.

However, their vibrant hues can also pose a risk to your smile. If you're a berry enthusiast, please take heed: Please be sure to rinse your mouth thoroughly with water after indulging in these delightful fruits.

This simple step helps minimize the risk of staining, allowing you to savor the goodness of berries while safeguarding your smile.

Sports Drinks Tough on Teeth? You Bet!

While sugary drinks can pose a threat to your dental health, some energy and sports drinks might be particularly damaging. Research published in General Dentistry reveals that these beverages, as well as bottled lemonade, can gradually erode tooth enamel. This erosion can result in teeth that are thin, translucent, and discolored. To protect your teeth from erosion:

- **Avoid Prolonged Sipping:** Try not to sip these drinks over an extended period.
- **Rinse with Water:** After consuming these beverages, rinse your mouth with water to help wash away harmful acids.

Sugary Drinks

We get it, saying goodbye to sugary drinks might not be your thing, but guess what? The American Dental Association has a sweet tip for you! Just by cutting down on those sugary sips and reaching for other tasty options, you're already winning! Water, unsweetened tea, milk, plain sparkling water, and even diluted juice are all fab choices with little or no sugar. So, why not swap out that sugary drink for one of these delightful picks? Your smile will thank you!

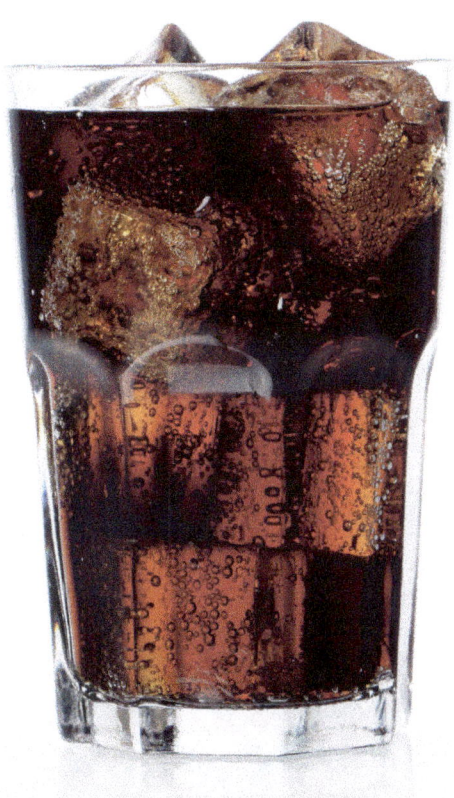

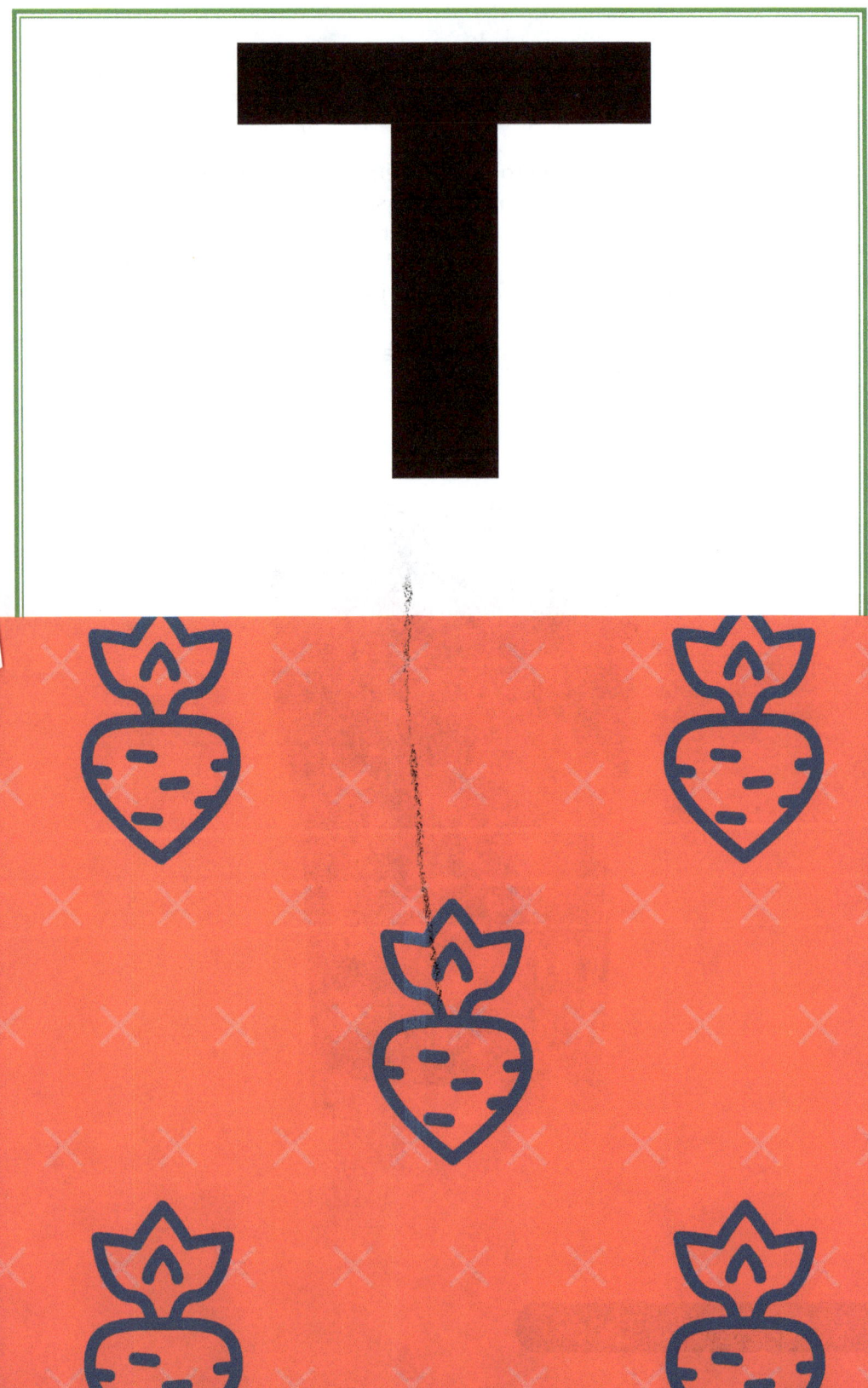

Turmeric

White Gold: Illuminating Your Smile with Turmeric!

Turmeric, known for its bright yellow color and powerful medicinal properties, is a surprising friend of teeth whitening. This spice contains cur cumin, a compound with anti-inflammatory and antimicrobial properties. According to a study published in the Journal of Contemporary Dental Practice, turmeric can help reduce plaque and gingivitis, making it a great addition to your oral care routine. Just keep in mind not to use it too generously.

How to use:
Mix a small amount of turmeric powder with water or coconut oil to form a paste.

Apply the paste to your teeth using a toothbrush.

Leave it on for a few minutes before rinsing thoroughly. With its vibrant golden hue, Turmeric isn't just a spice for culinary delights; it's also a natural whitening agent packed with potent properties.

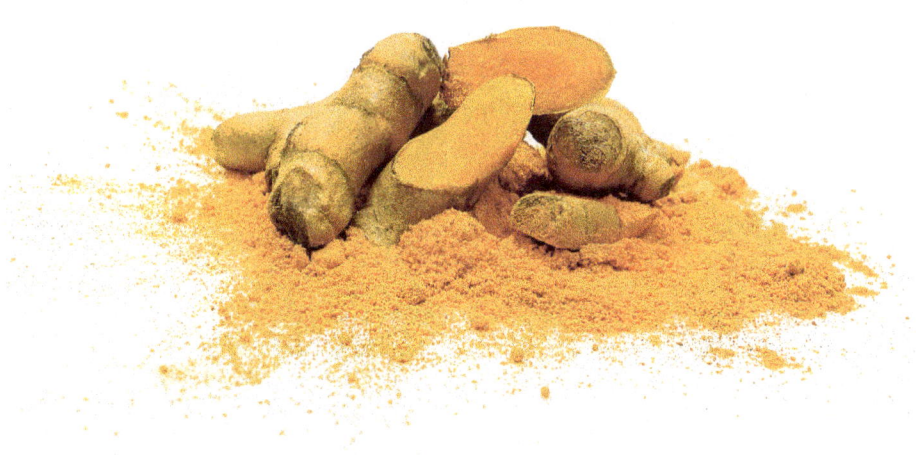

Tomatoes

A Juicy Secret for a Brighter Smile

Tomatoes are not only a versatile and tasty addition to your meals but also a natural aid for teeth whitening. Rich in vitamins C and A, tomatoes help strengthen enamel and support gum health. Their natural acidity assists in breaking down surface stains, while their high water content stimulates saliva production, which helps cleanse your teeth and wash away food particles. Enjoy tomatoes as part of your diet to enhance your oral care routine and achieve a naturally brighter, healthier smile!

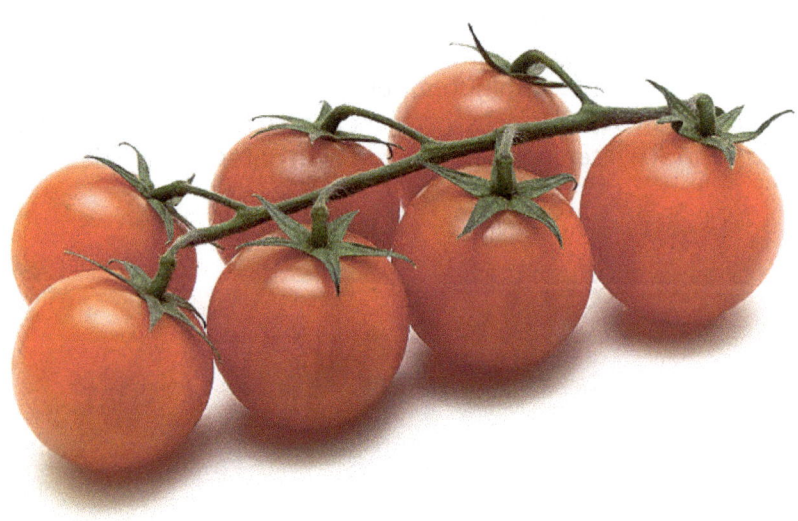

Turnips

A Root Veggie for a Brighter Smile

Turnips are not just a hearty root vegetable—they also support natural teeth whitening. Their crunchy texture helps gently scrub away food particles and plaque, reducing surface stains. Rich in vitamin C, turnips contribute to gum health and strengthen enamel. Additionally, their high water content stimulates saliva production, which aids in naturally cleansing your teeth. Incorporate turnips into your diet to enhance your oral care routine and enjoy a naturally brighter, healthier smile with this nutritious and versatile veggie.

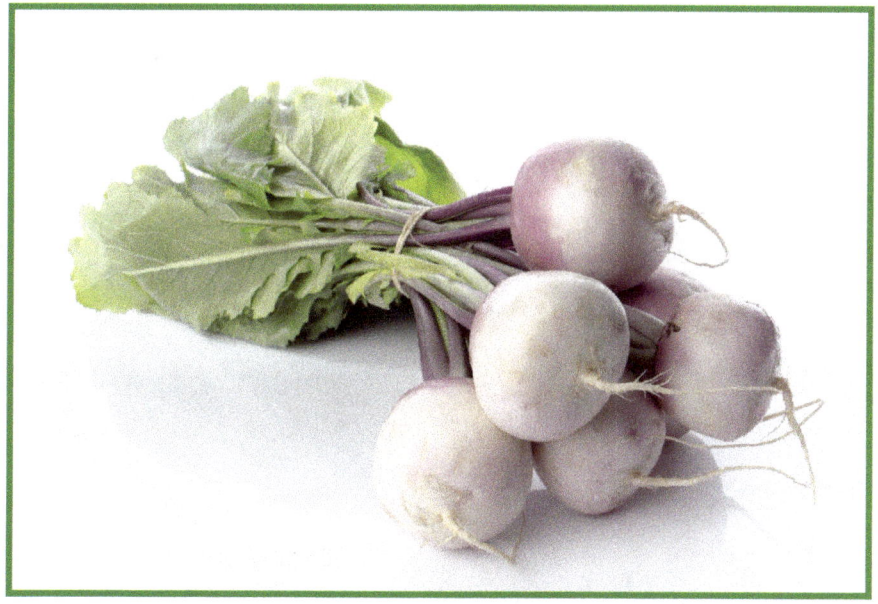

U

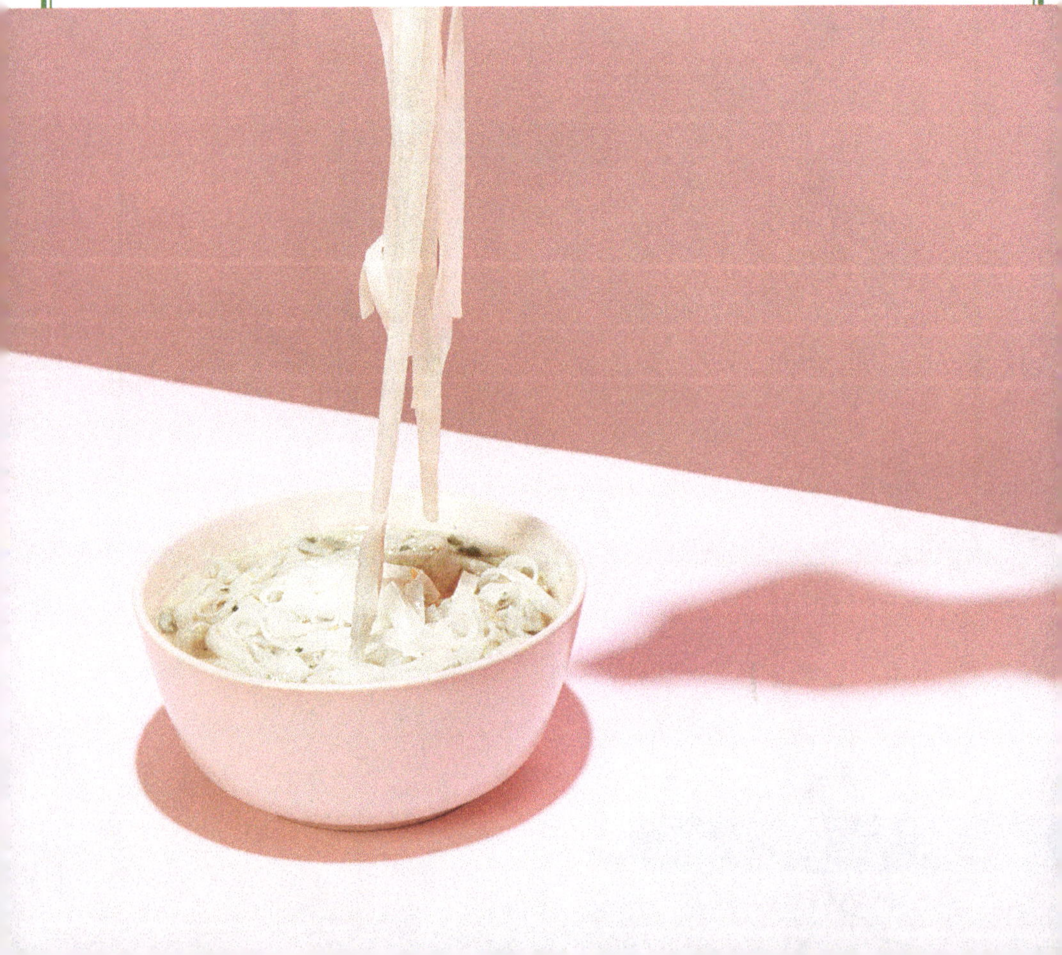

Udon Noodles

Although udon noodles may not have direct teeth-whitening properties, choosing whole-grain varieties can be a smart addition to a smilefriendly diet. These noodles offer essential nutrients that support overall oral health, contributing to strong gums and healthy teeth as part of a balanced diet.

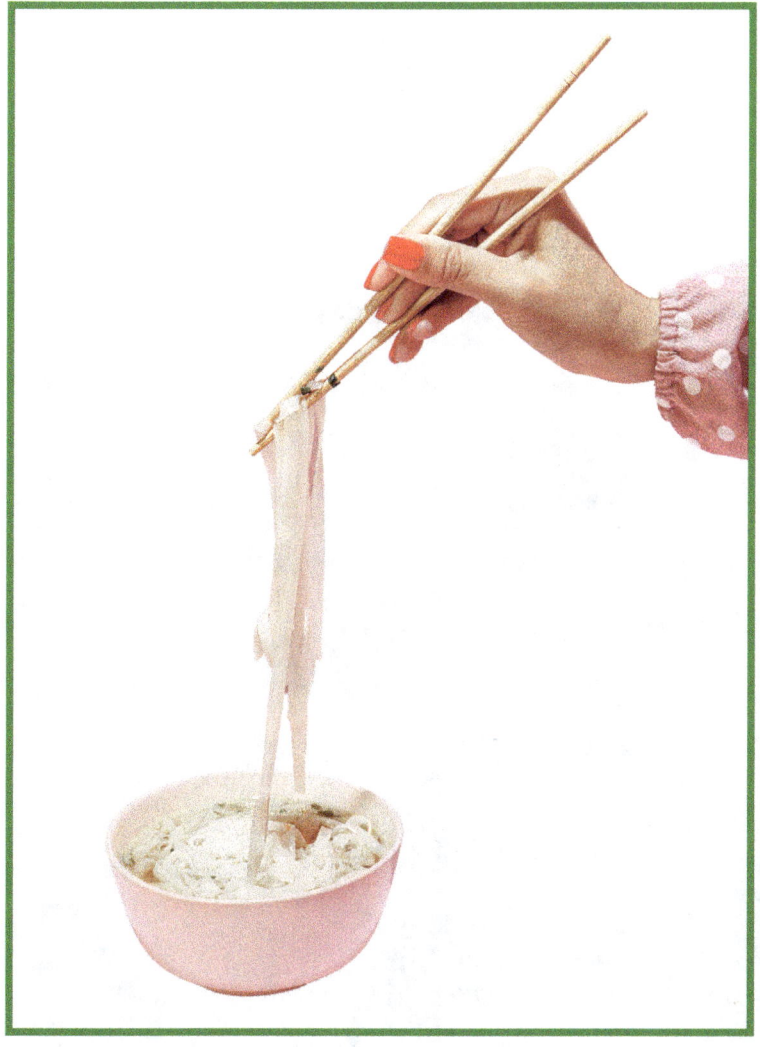

V

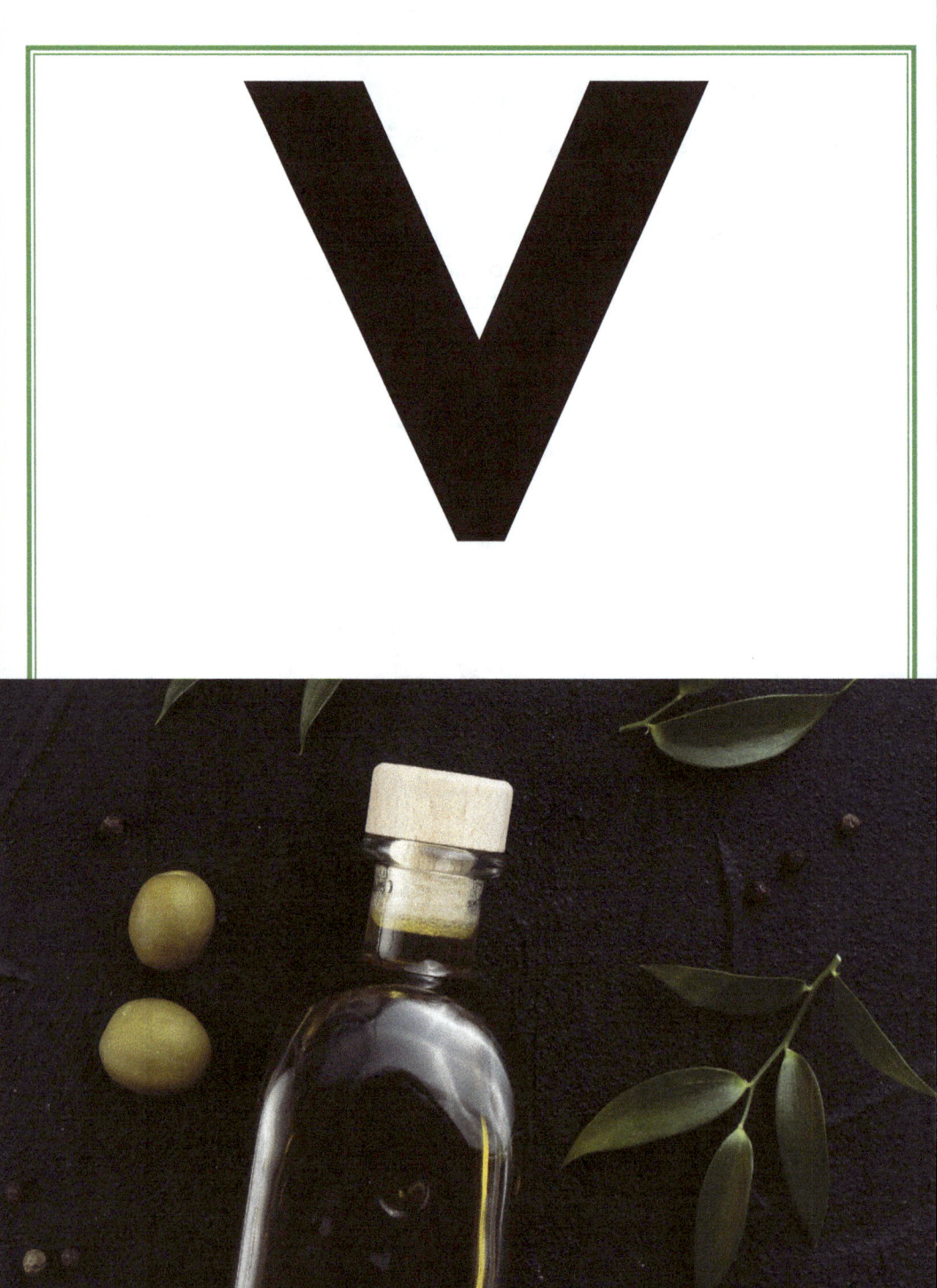

Extra Virgin Olive Oil

A Natural Aid for a Brighter, Healthier Smile

Extra virgin olive oil, renowned for its health benefits, can also play a role in promoting oral health and a brighter smile. Here's how it can benefit your teeth and gums:

1. **Natural Stain Remover:** The oil's natural properties help dissolve stains on the surface of teeth, contributing to a whiter appearance. Regularly swishing with olive oil can help lift superficial stains caused by foods and beverages.
2. **Promotes Gum Health:** Olive oil has anti-inflammatory properties that can help reduce gum inflammation and support overall gum health. It can be especially beneficial for people with sensitive gums or those prone to gingivitis.
3. **Antibacterial Properties:** Olive oil contains compounds that can help reduce harmful bacteria in the mouth, contributing to a healthier oral environment and reducing the risk of plaque buildup and cavities.
4. **Moisturizes Oral Tissues:** The oil helps keep the oral tissues hydrated, which can be particularly beneficial for individuals experiencing dry mouth. A well-lubricated mouth is essential for maintaining good oral health.
5. **Supports Enamel Health:** The fatty acids and antioxidants in olive oil can help protect tooth enamel from erosion, supporting strong and resilient teeth.

To incorporate extra virgin olive oil into your oral care routine, consider oil pulling—a practice of swishing oil in your mouth for about 15-20 minutes daily before brushing. This method can help promote oral hygiene and enhance your smile's brightness while supporting overall gum and teeth health.

W

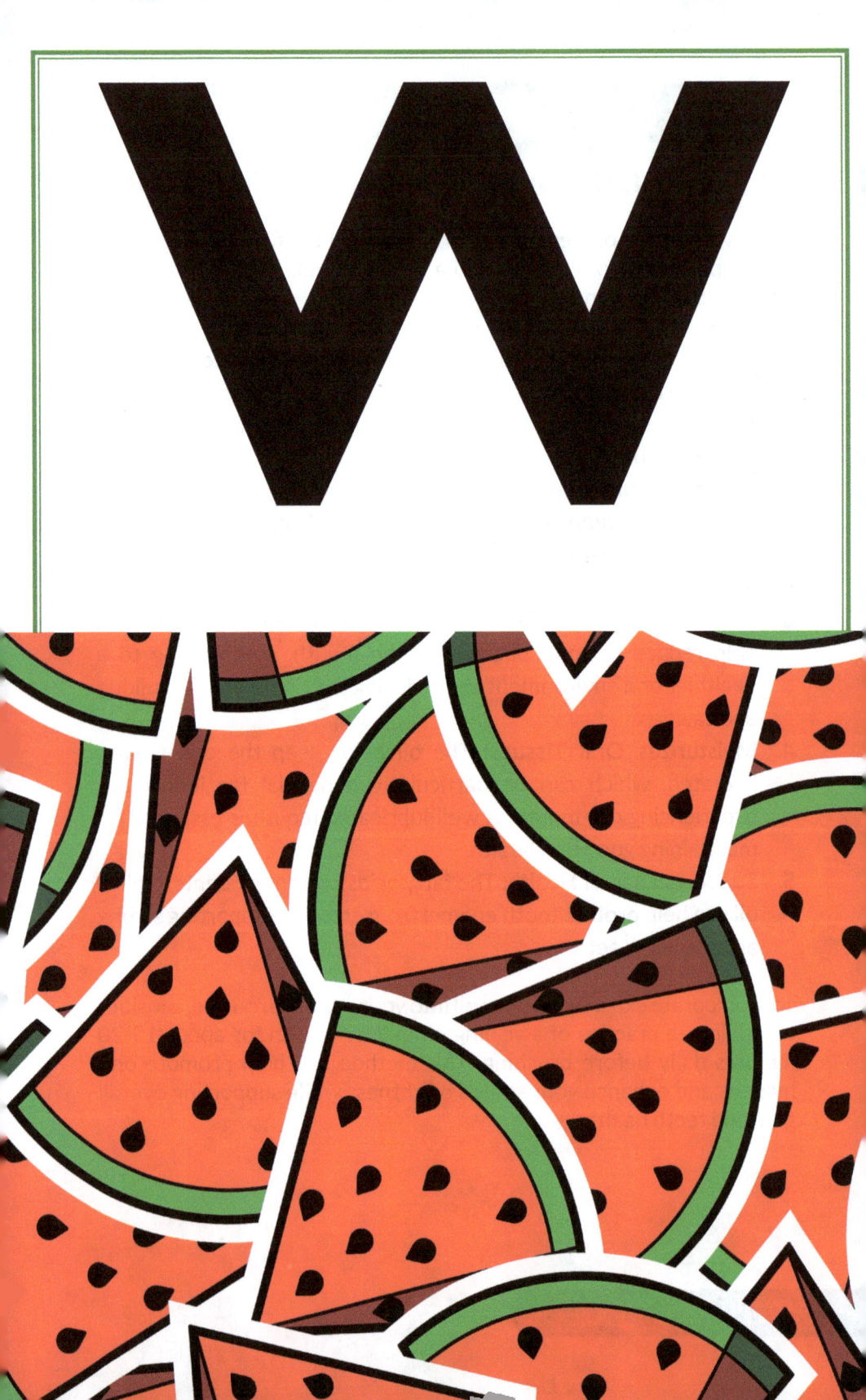

Walnuts

A Nutty Boost for a Brighter Smile

Walnuts are more than just a nutritious snack—they also aid in natural teeth whitening. Their unique texture provides a gentle abrasive action that helps remove surface stains and plaque buildup from your teeth. Rich in omega-3 fatty acids and antioxidants, walnuts support gum health and strengthen enamel. Additionally, their high fiber content promotes saliva production, which naturally cleanses your teeth and washes away food particles. Enjoy walnuts as a healthy addition to your diet to enhance your oral care routine and achieve a naturally brighter, healthier smile!

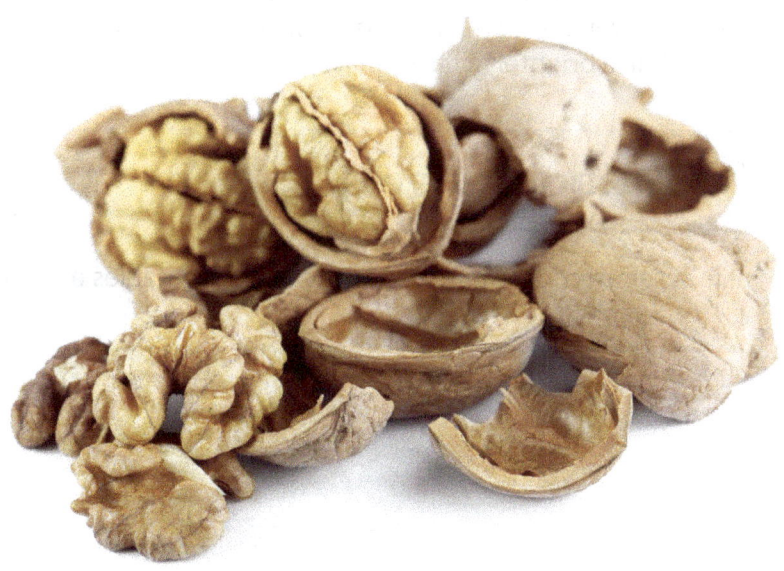

WATER

H2-Oh Yeah!

Discovering the Hydrating Benefits of a Dazzling Smile!

H_2O keeps you hydrated and smiling brightly. Sip and swish between glasses of wine and when eating dark, pigmented foods to prevent staining. Just be sure to drink still over sparkling: Bubbles can erode enamel and harm teeth.

Water works to reduce staining. Drink water with meals and rinse your mouth with water after eating. Just sip and give a final swish (and swallow) after a meal.

Drinking Water Helps Keep Your Teeth White

Water is a natural cleanser, rinsing away food particles after meals and between snacks. By drinking water, you help prevent stains from food and beverages, especially if you sip or rinse your mouth right after enjoying something that might cause discoloration. This simple habit helps maintain a brighter, whiter smile.

Nibble Knowledge

Sprinkle sesame seeds on salads and steamed vegetables a few times a week for a gentle tooth cleaning.

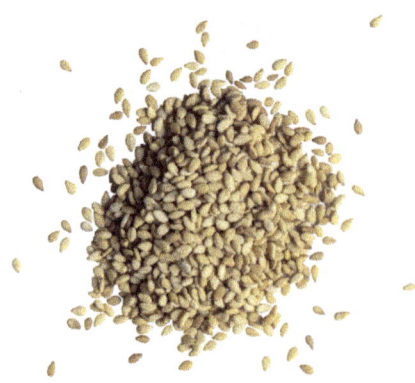

Watermelon

Juicy Secrets: Unveiling the Smile -Refreshing Benefits of Watermelon!

Watermelon is a refreshing summer treat, and it's also a natural teeth whitener! It contains more malic acid than strawberries.

It is also believed that the fibrous texture of watermelon scrubs your teeth, which helps remove stains.

Watermelon, packed with its abundance of water, serves as a natural hydrator for the mouth, promoting saliva production that aids in keeping it refreshed and free from debris.

Rich in vitamins A and C, it actively nurtures gum health. Additionally, the act of chewing watermelon naturally assists in cleansing the teeth.

Indulge in a refreshing slice of watermelon for its high water content and natural ability to promote saliva production. Saliva helps wash away food particles and bacteria, contributing to a brighter smile.

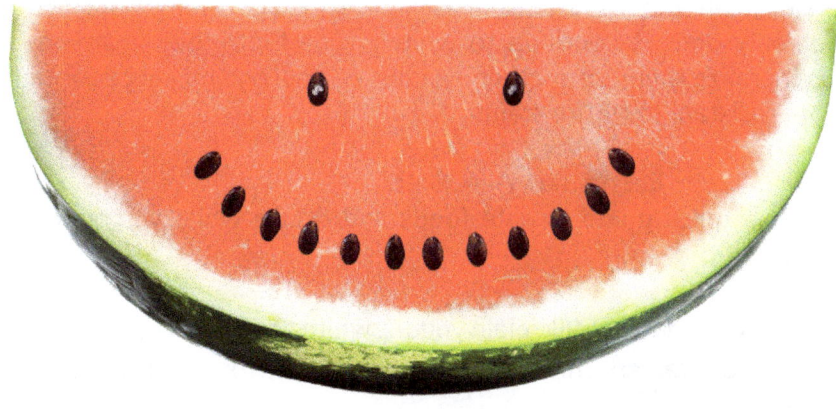

The White Diet: Essential Tips After Teeth Whitening

So, you've just achieved that dazzling, bright smile by whitening your smile with a home kit or at your dentist—congratulations! Now, how do you keep your teeth looking their absolute best? Enter the **White Diet,** a crucial step to maintain your stunning results and ensure your teeth stay white and healthy.

What is the White Diet?
The **White Diet** is a simple but effective eating plan to follow after teeth whitening. It involves sticking to foods and beverages that are light in color and avoiding those that can stain your freshly whitened teeth.Think of it as giving your smile the royal treatment it deserves!

Why is the White Diet Important?
After a whitening treatment, your teeth are especially porous and more prone to staining. This means that they can easily absorb colors from the foods and drinks you consume, which could dull your results if you're not careful. Following the **White Diet** helps protect your new smile and prolong the effects of your whitening treatment.

SmileSerum® – Your Whitening Ally
While the **White Diet** is key to maintaining your bright **smile, SmileSerum® by WhiteBrights®** adds an extra layer of protection. Not only does it continue to whiten your teeth, but it also helps remineralize them, strengthening your enamel and making your teeth more resistant to future stains.

What Can You Eat on the White Diet?
Here's a quick guide to safe foods and drinks while you're on the **White Diet:**

- **Dairy Products:** Milk, plain yogurt, white cheese
- **White Meats:** Chicken, turkey, and pork (preferably baked or grilled)
- **Vegetables:** Cauliflower, peeled potatoes, mushrooms
- **Pasta & Rice:** White pasta, white rice, and white bread

- **Beverages:** Water, milk, clear sodas

What to Avoid?

To keep your smile looking its brightest, steer clear of the following for at least 48 hours after whitening:

- **Dark Beverages:** Coffee, tea, red wine, cola
- **Colored Sauces:** Tomato sauce, soy sauce, balsamic vinegar
- **Brightly Colored Fruits:** Berries, cherries, grapes
- **Strongly Colored Spices:** Turmeric, paprika, curry powder

Final Thoughts

By sticking to the White Diet and using **SmileSerum®** regularly, you'll not only keep your teeth looking their best but also give them the care they need to stay strong and healthy. Remember, a little bit of effort now will go a long way in maintaining that stunning, bright smile you've worked so hard to achieve!

Remember to use code **SMILEDIET826** for 25% OFF at **www.WhiteBrights.com**.

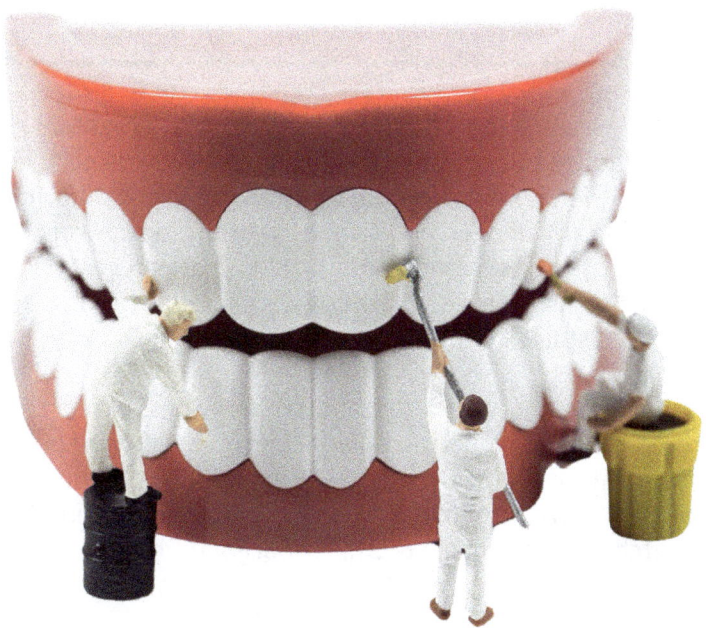

Wine

Uncorking Smiles

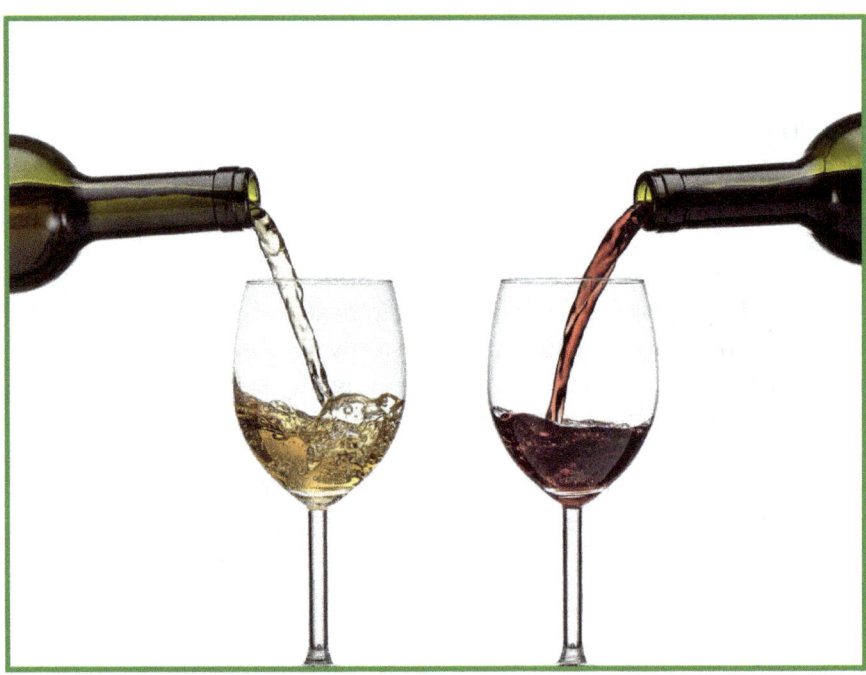

Unveiling the Grape Expectations of Wine for Your Brighter Grin

Savoring a glass or two of red wine can indeed provide certain health benefits. However, it's important to be aware of its potential impact on your smile. The chromogen and tannins present in red wine have the propensity to stain teeth and contain acids that can gradually erode your enamel. Consequently, this makes your teeth more susceptible to deep-seated stains from other foods and beverages.

It's worth noting that both red and white wines, when consumed excessively, can lead to teeth staining. Despite red wine being more notorious for its staining effects, the acidic nature of white wine can also cause concern. The acidic composition of white wine has been found to etch tiny grooves in teeth, rendering them more porous and susceptible to staining over time. As such, moderation and proper oral care are key to enjoying wine without compromising the brightness of your smile.

I will be the last one to ever suggest that you stop drinking wine. Here's a great tip for all you wine drinkers.

Red wine can naturally stain your teeth due to its deep, rich color. You can reduce its staining effect by drinking water alongside or after your wine, which will help rinse away compounds that could stain your teeth.

Additionally, if you are able, brushing your teeth about 30 minutes after consumption will help reduce the possibility of actual staining. Speaking of award-winning wines!

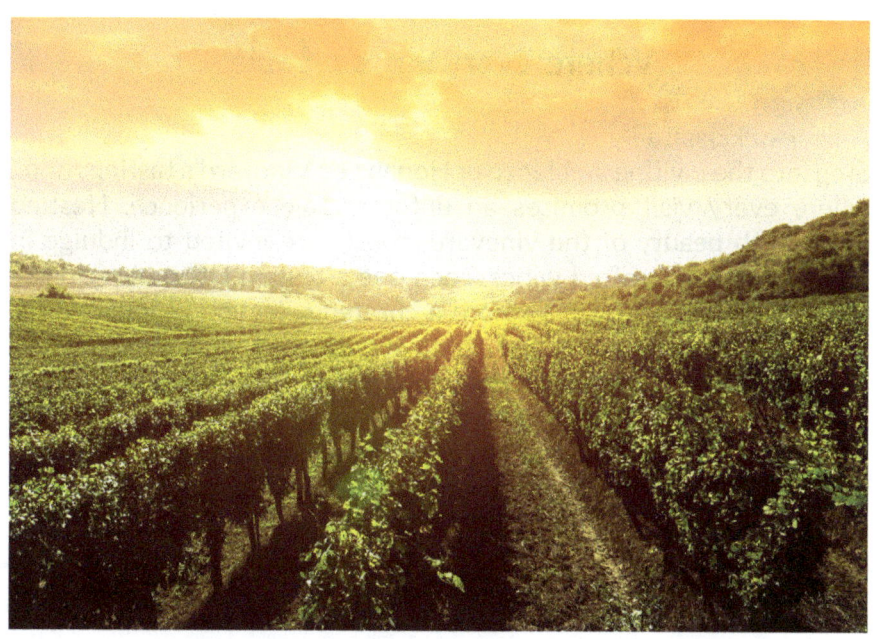

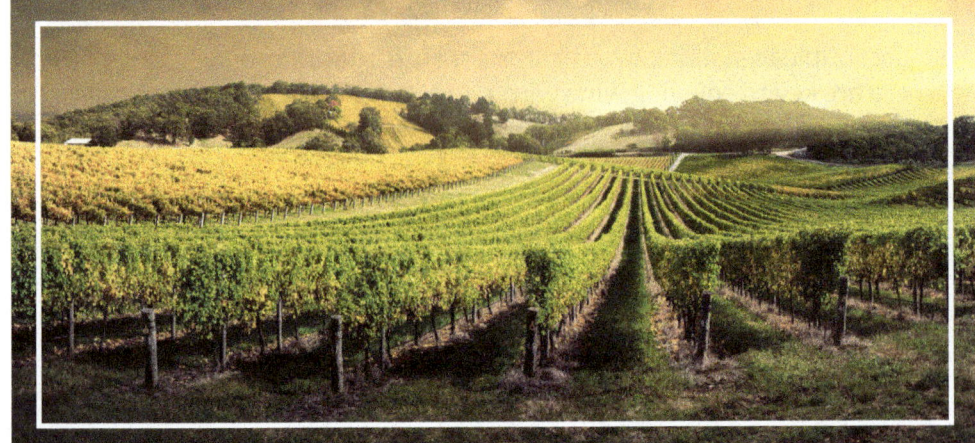

Special VIP Invitation

Honah Lee Vineyard
Gordonsville, VA

Where Every Sip is a Smile

A Taste of Hospitality
Step into the inviting ambiance of Honah Lee Vineyard's tasting room, where every visit promises an unforgettable experience. Nestled in the lush beauty of the vineyard, guests are invited to indulge in an array of handcrafted wines, each one a testament to the artistry of the winemaking craft. Explore a curated selection of local crafts, and artisanal jams and jellies, adding a touch of Virginia's culinary heritage to your visit. As well as wines, Honah Lee also offers Meads and Cider crafted beverages in the tasting room. A bit of something for everyone's tastes. Since its inception in 1992, my family-owned vineyard has been crafting award-winning wines that capture the essence of Virginia's wine country.

Join Us in Raising a Glass

Whether you're a seasoned oenophile or a curious novice, Honah Lee Vineyard welcomes you to embark on a journey of discovery through Virginia's rich winemaking tradition. From the vineyard to the tasting room, every moment spent at Honah Lee is infused with warmth, hospitality, and, above all, the joy of sharing exceptional wine with those who matter most. Experience the magic of Honah Lee Vineyard, where every sip is a smile. Tell them I sent you!

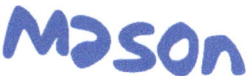

https://www.honahleevineyard.com

May we suggest, BrightenUp®

Keep your smile always prepared with these ultimate whitening deep cleansing teeth wipes. They are expertly crafted to eliminate surface films. Enriched with nourishing Vitamin E.

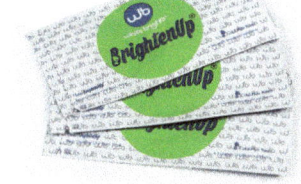

BrightenUp® can be found at
https://www.WhiteBrights.com

Y

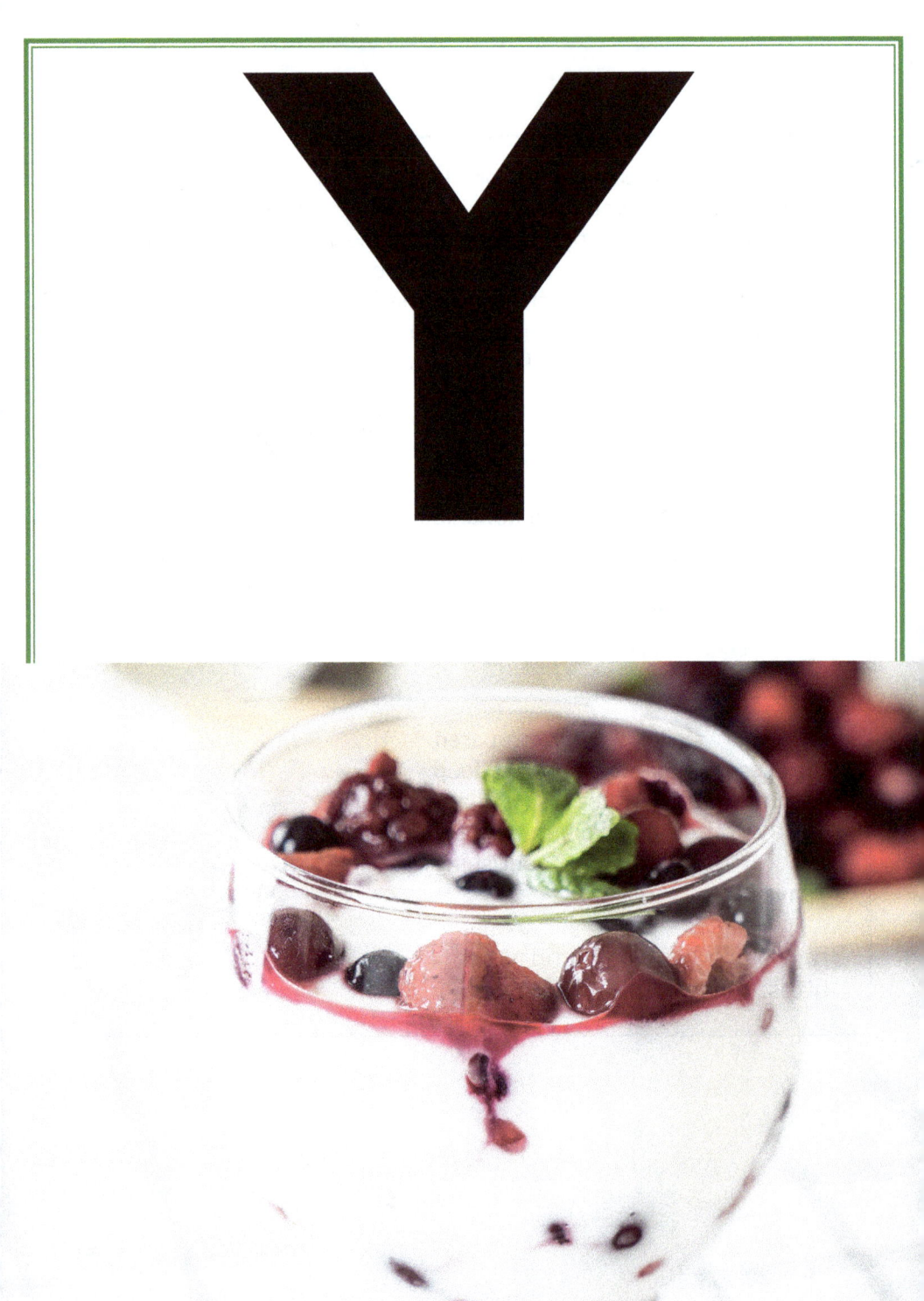

Yogurt

Explore the oral health benefits

Yogurt Yum: Unveiling the Creamy Delights for a Brighter Smile!
Bacteria buildup is a common culprit behind bad breath, plaque, and gum disease. Research suggests that incorporating 6 ounces of plain, sugar-free yogurt into your daily diet could be effective in combatting germs nestled between teeth. The beneficial bacteria found in yogurt may help counteract harmful ones in the mouth, promoting a healthier oral environment.

Interestingly, yogurt consumption has shown promise in reducing cavities, especially among children who may be less inclined to brush their teeth regularly.

For those seeking a touch of sweetness, consider stirring in honey to plain yogurt. Honey contains compounds that inhibit bacteria, offering an additional layer of oral health protection. Embrace yogurt as a delicious and nutritious addition to your diet, supporting not only your overall health but also the well-being of your teeth and gums.

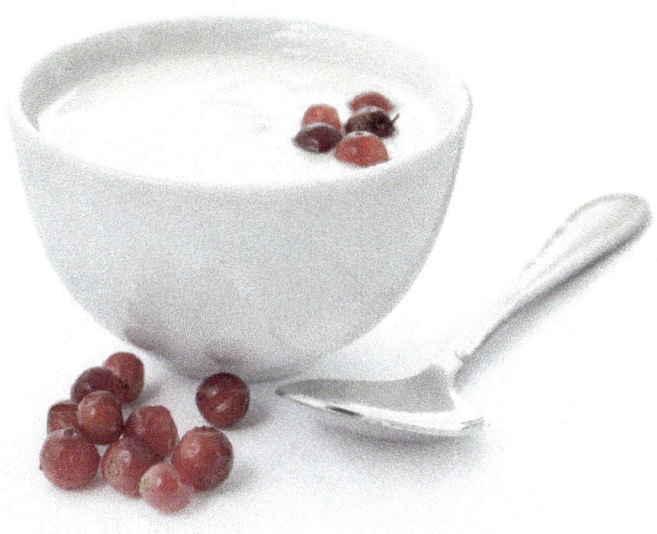

Z

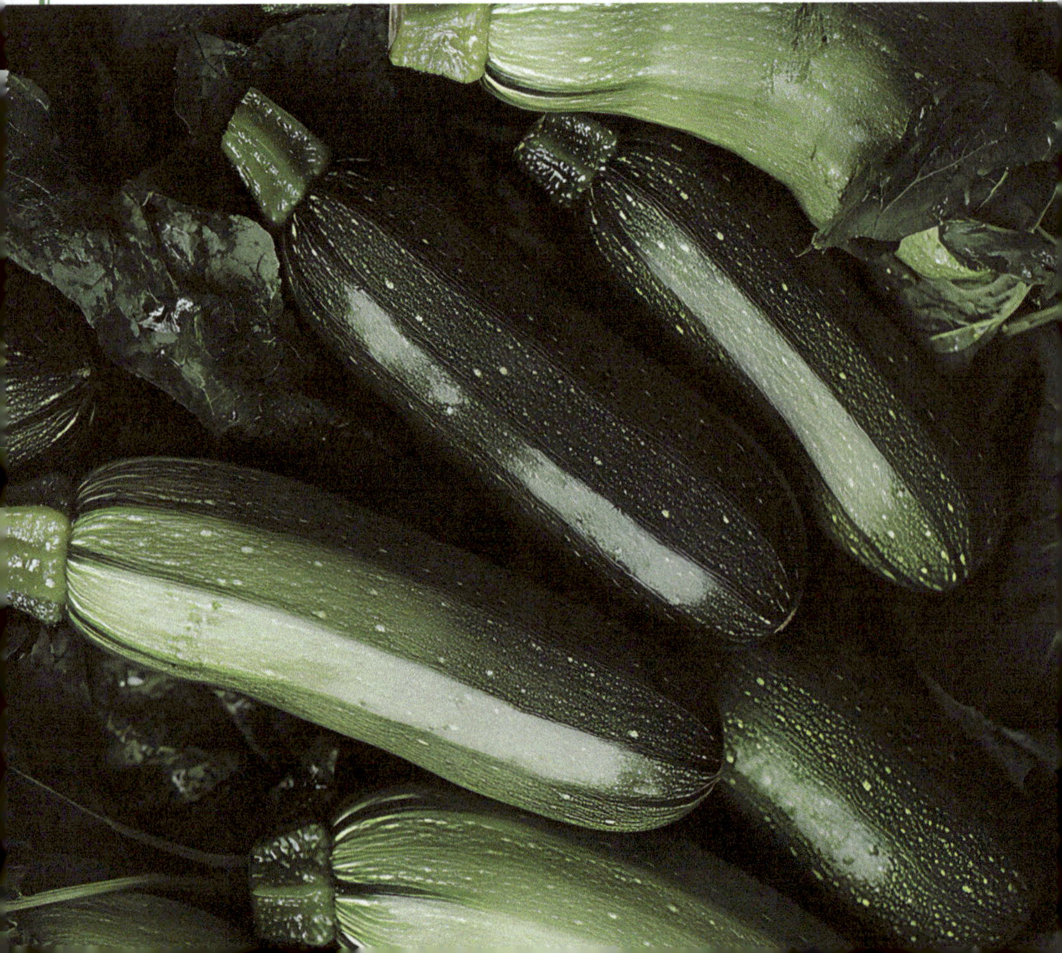

Zucchini

A Refreshing Ally for a Brighter Smile

Zucchini is more than just a versatile vegetable—it's a natural asset for teeth whitening. Its crisp texture helps gently scrub away surface stains and plaque buildup while boosting saliva production, which aids in cleansing your teeth. Rich in vitamins and minerals, zucchini supports overall oral health and helps maintain strong enamel. Enjoy zucchini in your meals for a tasty way to enhance your oral care routine and achieve a naturally brighter, healthier smile!

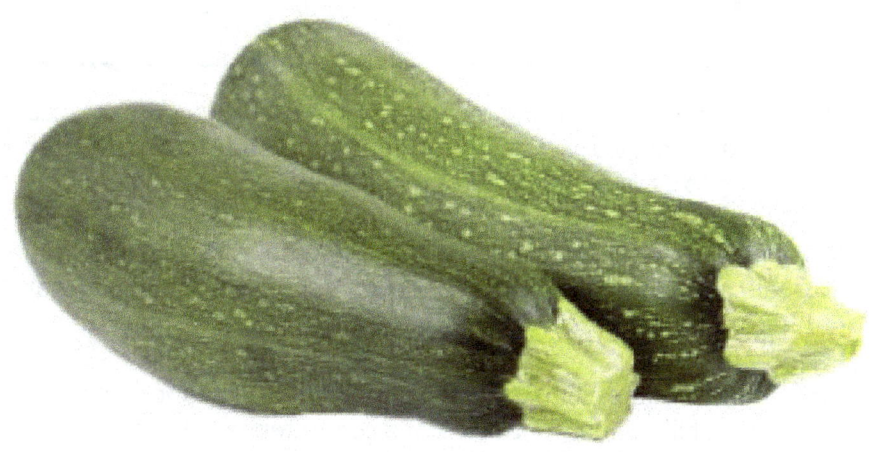

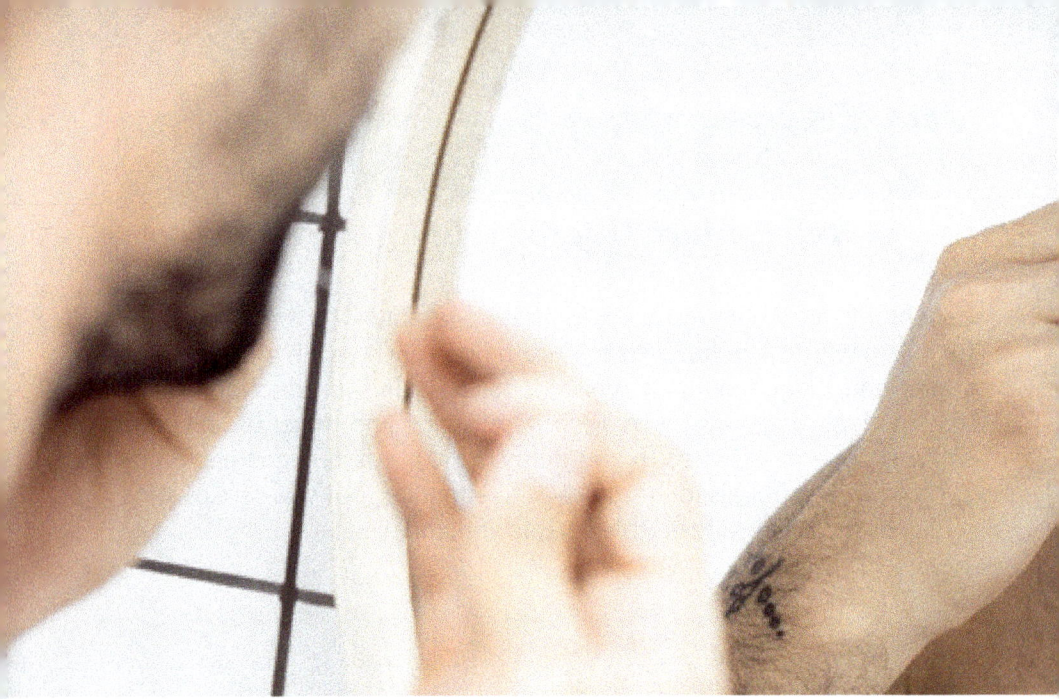

Why Embrace the Power of Smiling?

Smiling isn't merely a fleeting expression; it's a gateway to a cascade of feel-good chemicals like dopamine, serotonin, and endorphins, each contributing to a tapestry of health benefits.

From lowering blood pressure and boosting endurance to alleviating pain, reducing stress, and fortifying our immune system, the perks are plentiful.

What's more, studies illustrate how a smiling demeanor enhances perceptions of likability, politeness, and competence, often translating into heightened productivity. Beyond its impact, smiling possesses a contagious charm, stimulating neural pathways in others' brains, and prompting them to reciprocate with smiles of their own.

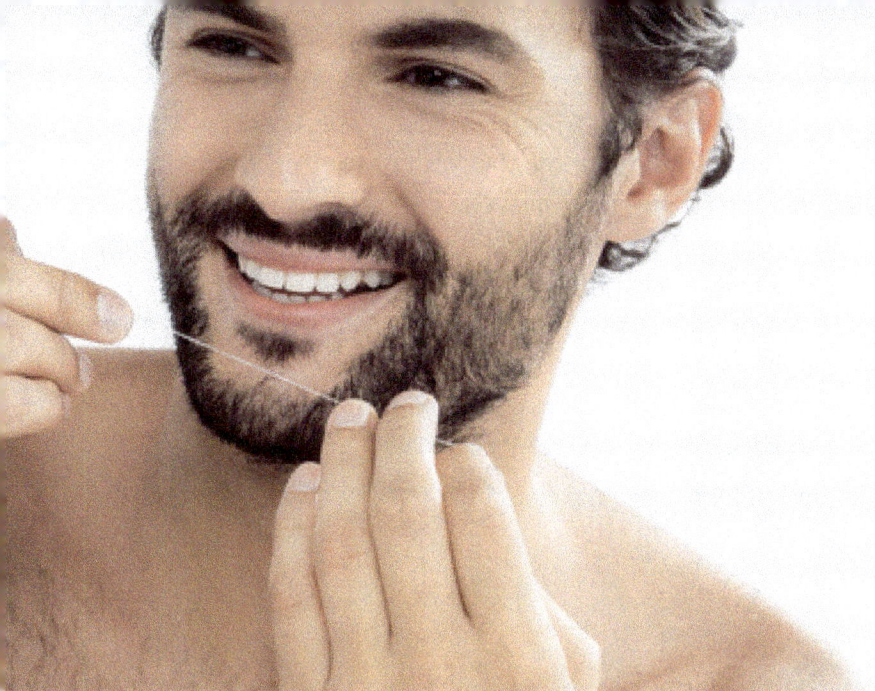

Try a Smile Challenge

Should you yearn to amplify your daily dose of smiles and reap the rewards of this simple yet profound gesture, why not initiate a daily ritual of gently coaxing those lips upward?

As you bask in the glow of your own smiles, here are three delightful smile challenges to infuse more joy into your life:

1. **The Post-It-Note Quest** – Arm yourself with ten vibrant Post-it notes and inscribe them with reminders of people, places, or things that make you smile.

Position them where they'll catch your eye each morning, kickstarting your day with a burst of positivity.

Even better yet! My friend Chance captures things that make him smile and keeps them on his smartphone.

2. **The Waiting Adventure** – Transform mundane moments of waiting, whether it be in traffic or at the checkout line, into opportunities to radiate warmth through a smile. Observe as your gesture kindles a chain reaction of smiles in those around you. There is no doubt, that smiles truly are contagious!
3. **The 19 Expedition** – Scientists have decoded a fascinating array of 19 smile variations. How many can you explore? Engage in a playful experiment with your reflection, crafting an assortment of smiles and discovering the nuances of each.

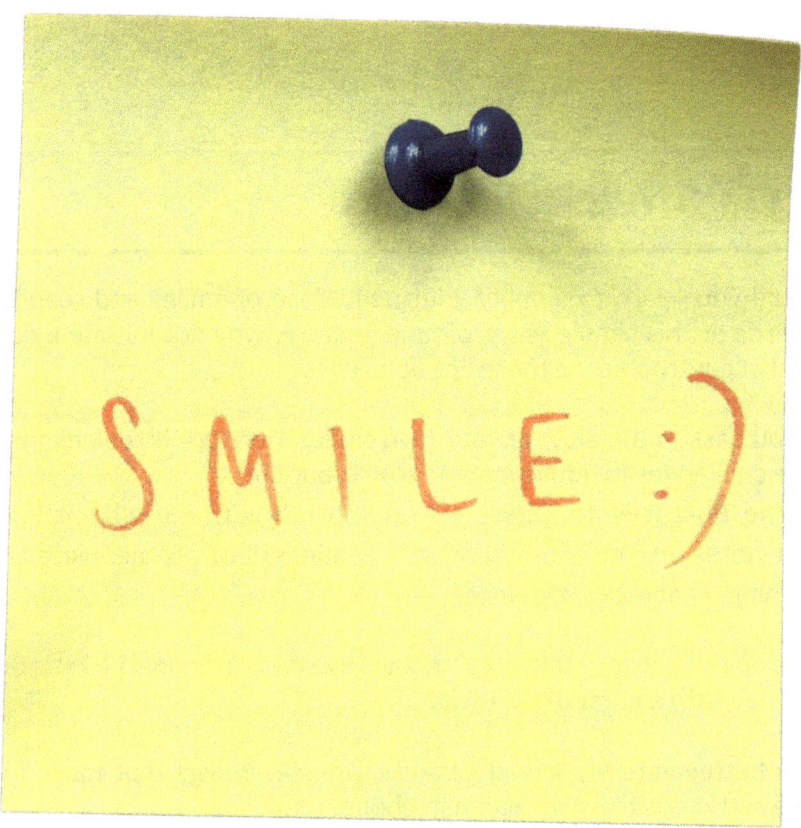

TIPS:

Pineapple and papaya have proteolytic enzymes that dissolve staincausing proteins on your teeth.

Be mindful! Those dealing with untreated acid reflux disease will often face teeth staining.

For these individuals, it is important to keep a keen watch on the shade of your smile. Each of our teeth whitening kits comes with a wonderfully crafted credit card-style teeth shade guide.

Every hue and tone has been meticulously chosen to reflect realism. What's more, they're translucent, allowing you to easily match your shade by simply holding the card up to your teeth and indulging in your newfound joy: smiling!

"Keep Things Moving!"
Minimize the risk of staining by ensuring foods and drinks don't linger around in your mouth longer than necessary. And, of course, always remember to chew thoroughly before swallowing.

Snack on nuts and seeds like almonds and sesame seeds for gentle exfoliation. Their texture can help remove surface stains, leaving your teeth looking whiter, brighter, and healthier.

Typically abrasive, lightly colored foods, like celery and carrots or even crunchy nuts and sesame seeds—nothing with dark pigments will help remove plaque naturally and can lighten the appearance of your teeth.

First, water is the absolute best thing you can drink to keep your smile healthy. Rinsing your mouth out when you first wake up can help keep white spots from appearing. Second, as mentioned above, milk can be a great way to fortify your enamel and reduce stains.

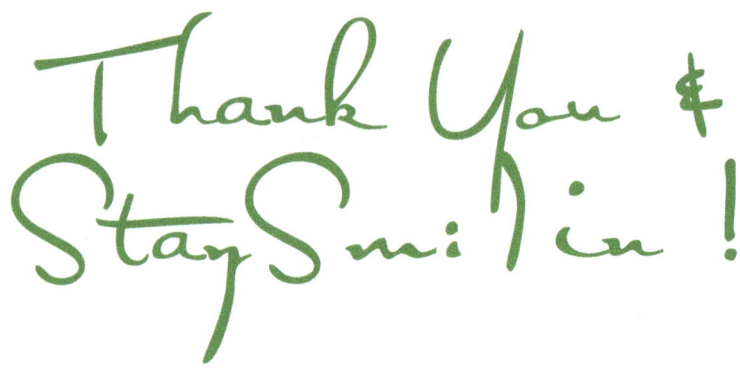

As you close the pages of The Smile Diet, remember that your journey to a whiter, brighter, and healthier smile is just beginning.

Embracing the foods that nurture your teeth and steering clear of those that dim your shine isn't just about following a diet; it's about adopting a lifestyle that celebrates your smile every day. Your teeth are more than tools for just chewing; they're the stars of your expressions, the gateway to your confidence, and a reflection of your overall health.

Stay committed to these simple, effective dietary choices, and you'll be rewarded with a smile that radiates positivity and well-being. At WhiteBrights®, we're thrilled to be part of your journey and are always here to support you with our innovative products and unwavering dedication to your smile's health and beauty.

Keep these tips in mind, stay smiling, and remember – the world is always a brighter place when you share your smile.

StaySm:)in', and best wishes for a lifetime of joyful, confident grins!

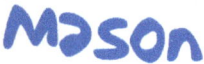

www.ingramcontent.com/pod-product-compliance
Lightning Source LLC
Chambersburg PA
CBHW060947050426
42337CB00052B/1637